Praise for
NOT ALL OF US ARE SAINTS

"In a beautifully clear and direct writing style, [Hilfiker] provides a riveting account of his experiences. . . . Writing in the vein of Jonathan Kozol and Alex Kotlowitz, Hilfiker's depiction of inner-city misery ought to stir the compassion of middle-class Americans and thereby inspire a deeper commitment to providing minimal health care."
—*Commonweal*

"Fascinating . . . Powerful . . . Hilfiker's is a stunning book for those exhausted by the health-care debate. It returns us, relentlessly and compellingly, to the problem that begot mandates, alliances, premium caps, and the rest: Many Americans don't receive decent medical care. . . . Toward the end, Hilfiker writes of the miraculous resolution of his long, seemingly impossible relationship with a chronic alcoholic named Clint Wooder. After months of detox, relapse, and mutual bitterness, the two men wordlessly celebrate Wooder's sobriety. It's hard to do these four paragraphs justice except to note that they constitute one of the most moving, joyous passages I've ever read—the finest moment in a deeply passionate account of what it is to be a doctor, and what it is to be poor."
—*Business Week*

"Hilfiker clarifies the nature of poverty and its awful power to break the human spirit. His plain-spoken account of his following the 'Mother Teresa Model' of poverty medicine radiates a certain nobility from which readers can draw hope and the recognition of humanity's oneness. An uncommon read."
—*Library Journal* (starred review)

*Please turn the page
for more reviews. . . .*

"Rarely have we been so powerfully forced to confront the plight of those who have been battered by homelessness, lack of education, poor nutrition, and addiction; rarely have we been made to see how grossly inhospitable to the spirit is poverty."
—*Publishers Weekly* (boxed review)

"A powerful report of the experiences of a physician living and practicing medicine in the inner city . . . This book is less about medicine than about class, race, and culture. . . . A deeply disturbing picture of the degradation of ghetto life and a painfully honest account of one man's attempt to do something about it."
—*Kirkus Reviews* (starred review)

"An important addition to the literature of contemporary life in the rich global power that the U.S. is."
—*Booklist*

"[A] testament to the small miracles that a small committed group can work."
—*Roanoke Times & World-News*

"Lucid . . . Compelling."
—*Readings: A Journal of Reviews and Commentary in Mental Health*

By David Hilfiker, M.D.:

HEALING THE WOUNDS: A Doctor Looks at His Work
NOT ALL OF US ARE SAINTS: A Doctor's Journey with
the Poor*

*Published by Ballantine Books

Books published by The Ballantine Publishing Group
are available at quantity discounts on bulk purchases
for premium, educational, fund-raising, and special
sales use. For details, please call 1-800-733-3000.

NOT ALL OF US ARE SAINTS

A Doctor's Journey with the Poor

David Hilfiker, M.D.

BALLANTINE BOOKS • NEW YORK

A version of Chapter 12, "Clint Wooder," appeared first in *Second Opinion* 18, no. 2 (October 1992): 43–53. *Second Opinion* is the journal of the Park Ridge Center for the Study of Health, Faith, and Ethics.

Library of Congress Catalog Card Number: 95-94962

ISBN 0-345-45975-X

This edition published by arrangement with Hill and Wang, a division of Farrar, Straus and Giroux, Inc.

Printed in the United States of America

To Janelle Goetcheus, M.D.

ACKNOWLEDGMENTS

Probably no book is ever written by one person alone, and this one—written over the course of almost ten years—is no exception; it is literally impossible for me to acknowledge each of the countless people who have contributed along the way.

Above all I am grateful to my patients—to the people of Belmont Street and to our guests at Christ House—who allowed me in various ways the privilege of sharing their lives. Their offerings of themselves, their trust in me, and their willingness to share with me are gifts I treasure. They are the inspiration for my writing.

The central ideas in this book evolved in the course of many conversations with staff and volunteers at Community of Hope Health Services, Columbia Road Health Services, and Christ House and were nurtured by members of Potter's House Church and other members of the Church of the Saviour community. While many will go unnamed, members of the Christ House mission group—Janelle and Allen Goetcheus, Don and Ellen Martin, Marcella Jordan, Loreta Jordan, and the late Mary Louise Norpel—along with the many volunteers in my Thursday morning small group at Christ House and the members of my classes in the Servant Leadership School provided an invaluable and ongoing sounding board for the themes explored here. Teresa Dyck and Midge Wholley, the nurses I worked with at Community of Hope, helped me more than they know to understand what it means to work compassionately with very poor people.

Many people read and commented upon the manuscript or portions of it in its many phases. Gordon Cosby's classes at the Servant Leadership School read the evolving manuscript and offered invaluable feedback while Diana Chambers did her best to keep class members from disseminating the book too widely. Gayle Boss, Newman Fair, Naomi Thiers, Sharon Martin, and others in the Writers' Group were tolerant of this nonpoet in their midst, patiently teaching me the difference between showing and telling. Rita Branham and Angela Robertson read the manuscript and gave me feedback from the points of view of people who have lived on Belmont Street and known these issues deeply and personally. Allen Holt and my sister Lois Kanter read the entire manuscript and offered suggestions and, more important, encouragement. As a scholar intimately familiar with the politics of poverty in this country, Jonathan Cobb read the manuscript in its early stages, offering invaluable advice.

Only an author can know how profoundly good editing shapes a manuscript-in-progress. If one is very fortunate, the book becomes through this shaping even more what the author originally intended rather than a compromise with "what will sell." I have been very fortunate. When this book was very rough, Tom Engelhardt grappled with its concepts (and with me), understood the essence of what I was about, and helped me over the course of many months articulate that essence. My editor at Hill and Wang, Sara Bershtel, and her assistant, Ariel Kaminer, meticulously reviewed every word and idea, further refining (and clearly improving) what is here. To them I am deeply grateful.

There are four women to whom I owe a particular debt of gratitude, without whom this book would not have been written. Janelle Goetcheus, M.D., first invited me to Washington to join her in the work she had initiated. Through our years working together as physicians, sharing the life of

Christ House, and struggling with the nature of poverty in Washington, D.C., she demonstrated to me what it meant to dedicate oneself to the poor for the love of God. Lois Wagner is my boss at Community of Hope Health Services, but she has been my soul mate on Belmont Street. We have leaned on each other in all sorts of practical ways, and she has shown me the reality of deep joy through relationships with the people of Belmont Street. Marianne Neisser, my psychotherapist and spiritual guide since 1984, taught me to reverence the brokenness within myself as deeply as Janelle and Lois taught me to reverence the brokenness of the poor. And my wife, Marja, through her own work teaching at the Academy of Hope, her welcoming of the poor into our own home, and her constant love, has kept before me the vision of a deeper life with the poor.

Finally, I must acknowledge my children, whose life with our guests at Christ House and with our friends at Joseph's House was ever an inspiration to me. They have sometimes suffered because of the decisions Marja and I made to live near the poor, but I am confident their lives are immeasurably richer. To them, and for them, I am grateful.

DAVID HILFIKER

CONTENTS

Chapter 1

A Doctor's Journey

This is absurd! What am I doing, near midnight, chasing John Turnell down the middle of Sixteenth Street? He's raving, swearing, pushing me away. What am I, a white man in white doctor clothes, doing entreating this drunken black homeless man to come home with me out of the night?

It was in October 1983 that John Turnell was first brought in from the streets. He could hardly walk. Buried in a dark, matted coat, pants reeking of urine, eyes cast on the floor, he sat passively in the corner of the examining room at Community of Hope Health Services.

"I hurt all over," he mumbled, barely audible. "My neck, my arm, my back, my leg. They're all achin'. My foot won't do nothin'."

He glanced up and our eyes met briefly. "I'm alcoholic," he said. "But I ain't had nothin' to drink in four days." He looked away. "Gotta stop these shakes. I know I gotta stop drinkin' this time. It's killin' me." He paused and I searched for something to say. But he began again, almost in a whisper. "And I'm pissin' all over myself, too. I can't stop it . . ." He hung his head. There was no expectation of help. He was simply reporting.

Thirty-eight then, he had jumped from a burning building six years earlier, breaking his back. "Pained ever since," he

1

said. He'd been hospitalized for surgery but got no relief
from his suffering.

I examined him. The pain, weakness, paralysis, and sen-
sory loss from his broken back and the concomitant nerve
damage were widespread. His left foot dragged, and the
large thigh muscles of his left leg had atrophied. The nerves
to his bladder were injured, so urine leaked all over his
clothing. He had lost sensation in his buttocks and could
not feel the large ulcers developing there that now drained
constantly.

He didn't have medical coverage, but the private hospital
at which I had privileges allowed me to admit an occasional
indigent patient for further examination. In the end, though,
there was not much to be done. Further surgery was not
recommended; long-term physical therapy would probably
have been of some help, but there was no way to pay for
it; the neurological damage—loss of sensation, constant
pain, foot drop, weakness, incontinence, impotence—was
permanent.

For the next several months, I saw John every week in
the clinic as I tended his ulcers. He stayed at a small shelter
in the neighborhood. His pain never really went away,
but—if he slept on a real bed and took pain medication
regularly—he could keep it under control. He got used to
wearing a leg bag for his urine. We found a foot brace so
he could walk without a limp. "It don't bother me so much
anymore," he said to me one day when I asked how he was
getting along. "You get used to it. I walk okay with the
brace, and at least I ain't pissin' all over. As long as I stay
sober, anyway," and he grinned.

I would see that grin again. It was big and bright, inviting, without a trace of resentment. And there was a certain
sparkle in the eyes that looked directly into mine. He
seemed to accept his wounds without anger or resignation.
I sometimes wondered how that was possible. Why didn't
he just give up the fight?

No, I exaggerate: He did not accept all his wounds . . .
not his impotence. "You know what it's like?" he would

say. "You know how she looks at you? She never says nothin', never gets mad. She says it don't make no difference to her, but when she's ready, no woman's gonna stay around for a man who can't perform." We once had a urologist ready to evaluate John's impotence, to look for something that could be done, but there was no insurance for the in-hospital tests, and the evaluation was put on hold . . . indefinitely, it turned out.

As John got better, the shamefaced, bedraggled derelict who came into my office every Thursday evening was gradually replaced by a handsome man with an engaging style. He looked me in the eye, smiled, made little jokes. He thanked me "for all you've done." I began to hope for his future. Abandoned as a child, alcoholic since adolescence, homeless for years, even *he* started to talk about a future. He got a custodial job nights, running a waxing machine. But then, a few weeks later, he told me his back had started acting up and he had quit the job. At my urging and with the help of our social worker, he applied for disability coverage under the Supplemental Security Program (SSI) of the federal Social Security Act, but he was not enthusiastic. He wanted to work, he said, not live off welfare.

Then, suddenly, John disappeared. I heard he was on the streets again. Several months later, his SSI disability claim was denied; the form letter said John was not sufficiently incapacitated! A volunteer lawyer associated with our clinic began an appeal, but John needed to appear in person, and no one knew where he was. The deadline passed.

When, after eight months, John finally showed up again at the clinic, I hardly recognized him. He was unshaven, gaunt; his lusterless eyes sagged in a hollow face. He moved slowly, agonizingly. Light reflected off the spittle in his beard. Sitting in the chair opposite me, he looked much smaller than his six feet. His dark, oversized clothes stank of urine, and his eyes remained fixed on the ground in visible shame. Although sober that evening, he had, he told me, started drinking again shortly after leaving his job waxing floors. Sleeping in alleys, stairwells, and crowded shel-

ters, he had aggravated his back pain, broken open the
ulcers on his buttocks, and lost both leg bag and foot brace.
Like a perverse safety alarm, however, the increasing pain
had put an end to the drinking and goaded him into the
clinic, embarrassed and repentant. I did not guess then how
often this pattern was to repeat itself.

We saw each other irregularly. He was always sober by
the time he showed up at the clinic. The pattern became unmistakable: He would begin to feel good about himself,
find a job, only to leave it after a few weeks (often because
it aggravated his back), and then disappear into the streets
and the alcohol. Invariably, as he got closer to indepen-
dence, some inner compulsion would shatter his dream.

As I watched him try to work while in severe pain, as I
noticed the cycle that always ended in the streets, I began
to encourage him not to work, to accept his disability. He,
however, was impatient. I tried again to help him get SSI
(which would at least allow him access to Medicaid and decent medical care), but the examiners turned him down
once more.

One autumn, three years after our initial meeting, John
returned, and I convinced him to move into Christ House,
the medical recovery shelter for homeless men that a group
of us had recently established with the help of our church
community. Better equipped and more intensively staffed
than the other shelters, dedicated exclusively to the care of
those who were too sick to be on the streets, Christ House
was also my home, where our family lived with a small
community of physicians, other staff people, and their families. Over many months with us, John maintained his sobriety, went through a twenty-eight-day, inpatient alcohol
treatment program, attended Alcoholics Anonymous
meetings daily, healed his buttock ulcers, strengthened his
foot, began managing his incontinence with special medications, and was able to keep even the constant pain to a tolerable level. He began attending classes at my wife Marja's
small adult education school, looking to get his high-

school-equivalency diploma. I allowed myself to hope again.

"I know it now: I just can't drink anymore, David . . . ever. It's killin' me. I'm alcoholic. I didn't like it when you sent me to that treatment program, but I understand now. I got to stay away from my friends on the street who drink. Got to get new friends. Y'all have helped me so much here, and I'm gonna make it this time. God has been good. You'll see. I'll get my GED, get a job, maybe get married. I'm gonna make it."

John "graduated" to a group home, continued attending GED classes with Marja, and was looking for work. Marja gave him one of our old family bicycles, so he could get around town. I felt proud of him. Then, once again, he disappeared. Two weeks later I was at the clinic when Sister Lenora Benda, the nurse in charge at Christ House, called. "John's back, David. He's been drinking, and he seems pretty depressed. He says he tried to swerve his bicycle into the path of a bus this morning, but the bus stopped. He keeps saying he wants to kill himself."

I sigh and am silent. Some small part of me is dying. I knew enough to expect it, to prepare for it, but I'm still not ready. Drunk again, and now suicidal! Is this real or some bizarre gesture? Where in this city will I find a psychiatrist to evaluate a homeless drunk? Even if we can get him help, will he get something more than the superficial consultation to which the homeless are so often limited?

"Can you get him over to St. Elizabeth's for a psychiatric evaluation, Lenora?"

"I think so. I think he still trusts me enough to let me take him."

Lenora manages to thread John through the system—an accomplishment in itself—and, that same afternoon, a psychiatrist at St. Elizabeth's, Washington's only public psychiatric hospital, evaluates John. The psychiatrist declines to hospitalize him, however, because the suicide attempt seems to her most likely to have been just a gesture brought on by his intoxication. John is released with instructions to make an appointment with me at the office.

The next evening, as I am lecturing to family physicians at their local professional association about the health care needs of the homeless in our city, the shrill signal of my pager interrupts. It seems that John has returned to Christ House and is uncontrollable. He's been marching back and forth, in and out of Christ House, lying down in front of traffic in Columbia Road or yelling and creating havoc inside. Could I come back and deal with John?

I return and try to slip upstairs to drop off my lecture notes and take a few moments to collect myself. Entering our apartment, I discover John in our living room talking with Marja. He's still drunk. "Dr. Hilfiker," he says, slurring his words, "don't send me over to St. Elizabeth's again. I'll be good, I promise. I don't need no hospital. I just need to stop drinking."

"But, John, what's this about running into the traffic, about committing suicide? I'm afraid you're going to hurt yourself. What's going to happen if a truck hits you?"

"Who told you I ran out into the street? Who said anything about suicide?" His usually quiet, reserved speech is loud and brassy. He eyes me belligerently, purses his lips, and pouts. "They're a goddamn liar. Why would I want to commit suicide? I didn't run out in no goddamn street."

Oddly, in my three years of working with John, I've not actually seen him drunk before. He has always been gentle, even embarrassingly obsequious; so his belligerence tonight catches me off guard. I have also not known him to lie. Has he forgotten his suicidal gestures? Suddenly he's whining again. "Please don't send me over to St. E.'s, Dr. Hilfiker."

I feel overwhelmed, boxed in. I wanted to be John's "friend," to lower the barriers between black and white, rich and poor. But now, in his extremity, he seems more like an alien, a drunk who has invaded my home. Will he turn violent? Will he try to stay? One part of me regrets my invitation to friendship and wants just to push him out to fend for himself. But another knows that without intervention John will disappear into the wilderness of the streets for another six months. And that is not the only conflict I find within my splintered thoughts and feelings. A wiser self knows that I am not in charge of John's recovery, that he must be the one to fight for sobriety; but I cannot let go. Frantically, I try to formulate even a short-term plan to return John to his path of recovery. But now he's up and pacing. I turn my back briefly, and he lurches from the apartment. For a moment I consider just letting him go. But I follow and finally catch up to him on the busy Columbia Road sidewalk outside our building. "Where are you going?" I take his arm softly. I'm self-conscious out here on the street, a white man pulling this unwilling black man through a sea of mostly colored humanity. "I ain't goin' to no St. E.'s, I can tell you that. I ain't goin' to no place like that. They just fuck you over." Despite his protestations, John allows me to lead him back into Christ House. He sprawls in a chair just across from the nurses' station, his long legs purposely obstructing even the wide main hallway.

I don't know what to do. We are not a detox center, and it's not fair to ask the lone night nurse and his aide to devote their entire energies to one patient withdrawing from alcohol; but I can think of no alternative. "John, do you want to spend the night here at Christ House?" I ask, bending our rules almost backward, partly because John has become in some sense a friend, mostly because I cannot admit that we have lost him this time around.

John agrees to take a tranquilizer to smooth the process of detoxification and lessen the likelihood of seizures, and I retreat to the nurses' station to write orders for his admission. Three times within the next fifteen minutes, however, John bolts from Christ House, and I run to retrieve him. Each time he's more belligerent; each time I am, perhaps, a little more hesitant to chase him.

I begin to fill out commitment papers, more out of despair than hope. As I finish, John once more runs outside, and I, once again, follow. As usual, Columbia Road is busy in the late evening: Latin music blares from small knots of Salvadoran men; the sidewalk café of the Ethiopian restaurant next door is full of black people laughing and talking in foreign tongues; well-dressed couples walk past beggars; children from a nearby housing development twist their way through the crowded streets even near midnight. Wading into this human sea, I catch up with John, but this time he is not about to be turned around.

"No way I'm goin' to St. E.'s. I thought you was my friend, Dr. Hilfiker. You ain't my friend." He stares straight forward and marches on, shouting epithets at me as I trail behind. "You just like all those other white motherfuckers. You don't care for no niggers. You get paid all that money to take care of us. We don't get nothin'."

I follow along in silence for almost a mile. What am I doing here, well past any reasonable bedtime, chasing a drunk down this street? Finally I stop and call to him. "John, I'm going back. I want you to come with me."

He continues walking, but fifty feet later turns. We stare at each other for a full minute. Finally his tall body wilts like a limp doll's, and he drags himself back toward me, defeated.

I have no idea why he's changed his mind. Perhaps it is the residue of the trust I thought had bonded us over these years. Perhaps he simply feels powerless and enraged. Trying to start a conversation, any conversation, to keep John's mind off St. E.'s, I ask him whether he ever thinks about going back home, to the South. "I never knew my mother," he says, apparently answering some question of his own. "She was crazy, spent most of her days in the state hospital. 'Paranoid schizophrenic,' they called it. My father, he drank a lot. I never saw him till I was six, and he came back home just to beat me. He kept telling me I was bad, just like her. He said I was crazy, too, and belonged in a hospital just like her. He hated me. Never said nothin' good about me. I lived at different places, but mostly I just raised myself. I started drinkin' when I was twelve. I knew I had found something there. It made me feel good. When I drink, I ain't afraid to say nothin'. When I'm sober I can't say what's on my mind. I couldn't tell you any of this if I wasn't drinkin'." I have learned more about John's past in these two minutes on the street than in two years of interviews. He looks at me and grins . . . that wide smile with those white teeth almost luminous against the dark night . . . but fear lies behind the eyes.

Back at Christ House sometime around midnight, I put John into a room and continue the process of committing him for psychiatric help. First, I call the public Crisis Resolution Unit, which is specifically mandated to intervene in situations like this. The receptionist says they are currently "short-staffed" and won't be able to help. She suggests calling the police. The police dispatcher says a unit will be "right over." When—after half an hour—nothing happens and I can hear John getting restless, I call again. "Well, you didn't say it was an emergency," the dispatcher says testily. Ten minutes later, John runs from his room. I catch up with him for what feels like the tenth time just as he lurches into the street and sprawls in front of an automobile, which jerks to a halt.

A moment later a squad car pulls up. I explain the situation to the officer and show him the commitment papers I have completed. The officer looks troubled. He tells me the police are not allowed to transport psychiatric patients from a "private facility" unless the police officer himself witnesses the patient being a danger to self or others. He says he didn't see John lying in the street. We will have to find our own transportation.

How could he not have seen John lying in the street? I can't believe it!

Asking the officer to wait, I call Crisis again. The head of the unit confirms my understanding that once I have filled out appropriate forms the police are obliged to transport. He asks me to wait a few minutes while he calls the precinct captain to straighten matters out. The officer and I wait. John goes into his room and passes out. I call Crisis back. They are still "working on it." Well after one o'clock in the morning, the officer leaves, John lies passed out in a room, and I go upstairs to bed. No one ever calls back from Crisis.

I'm not surprised to be awakened the next morning by the night nurse reporting that John has left.

Later that morning, Lenora calls me at the clinic. John has returned to Christ House, she has called Crisis, and this time a team has come and taken him to St. Elizabeth's. She asks me to call a certain psychiatrist at St. E.'s.

"Dr. Hilfiker, I have just examined Mr. Turnell," reports the doctor. "I feel that his suicide gestures are really the result of his drinking. I don't think that he requires mental hospitalization but rather alcohol detoxification."

I notice my hands shaking as I grip the telephone. "Doctor, John's suicide attempts are *obviously* caused by his drinking, but he's nevertheless a danger to himself at this time. As you know, they won't be able to *force* John to stay at the detox unit. He'll just walk out of there."

Despite my protests, the psychiatrist refuses to hospitalize John, referring him instead to the detox unit. John promptly walks out.

Over the next year John returns to my office several times. He no longer needs to wait until he is sober to visit. At one point he steals $250 from Angela, our receptionist. He marries a Haitian refugee with a two-year-old child. At the time of their wedding, he has known her just a month and has been drunk—as far as I can tell—the entire time. Just before the wedding, John comes, drunk, to my office with his prospective wife and child. While in our waiting room John starts hitting the boy, threatening to kill him. We eventually have to call Child Protective Services just to protect the boy. Since then I have seen John and his family several times on the street, he always walking fifteen feet ahead, she dragging the child behind, like a scene from an old foreign film.

* * *

I am a family physician who practices in Washington, D.C., a city replete with the most advanced medical technology in the world. But the reader who hopes to encounter clever medical sleuthing, rare cures, dramatic surgical interventions, or even a glimpse of the medical wizards who perform such heroics might as well close the book here. For I practice "poverty medicine," a profession more like the medicine practiced in the Third World than what is ordinarily considered "modern medicine."

Since 1983 I have worked at Community of Hope Health Services, a small, church-sponsored clinic in the inner city, and since 1985 also at Christ House, a thirty-four-bed medical recovery shelter for homeless men too sick to be on the streets yet not sick enough to be in the hospital. The medicine I now practice looks very different from what I did during the first seven years of my career, when I was a country doctor in a small town in northeastern Minnesota. There in Minnesota, the reassuring model of traditional medicine I had learned in my medical training still obtained: While other aspects of the patient's life were certainly important, illness was a distinct phenomenon that could basically be treated in and of itself. As "the Doctor" I assumed a role of real importance. My scientific medical expertise was useful, valued.

As soon as I entered the world of the inner-city poor, however, my "power" as a physician succumbed to the same forces that dominate the lives of my patients, and I had to learn what is really a new specialty—poverty medicine. I did not understand at first, but poverty medicine is in a sense about everything *but* medicine, about everything but doctoring as it is normally experienced in the middle- and upper-class world in which I was reared, trained, and first practiced. Disease as usually defined by medicine is prevalent and, by and large, worse among the poor of the inner city than among the more affluent. But health, in the world of my patients, is not simply a matter of disease and treatment; indeed the "strictly medical" is not the crucial factor in most healing.

By the very nature of my patients' circumstances, much of my work does not even feel like the proper use of my training and abilities. I spend my time listening to stories about shelter conditions, dangerous neighborhoods, economic hardship, family tragedies that I can do nothing about . . . except listen and care. I spend other large blocks of time *finagling* treatments for which another doctor would simply write a prescription: finding free medications, urging a specialist to volunteer care, traipsing by telephone through the maze of the public hospital to secure the results of a single test. Even in my day-to-day work, I am a "clinic doctor," dispensing routine medical care that—as far as the science of it is concerned—someone with far less education and experience could easily do.

Poverty medicine, of course, isn't recognized as a field within the profession of medicine. It's a medical specialty without schools, standards, accreditation, journals, or associations. Its few practitioners frequently do their own fundraising and band together for support in loosely knit alternative organizations without funding or power. It's a specialty with an enormous population of patients in America, yet virtually no practitioners.

Like my specialty, this book is, in a sense, about everything but medicine, for in working with people of poverty the simplest medical act reveals the deepest social contradiction.

This book is less about medicine than about class. My wife, Marja, and I are solidly middle-class. As a physician I could easily command a salary in excess of $100,000; as even a beginning teacher Marja could earn more than $27,000. Everything about our lives—our upbringing, our education, our level of consumption, the vacations we take, the church we attend, our prejudices about who deserves what and why—is deeply rooted in the middle class. This book explores what it is like for a middle-class doctor to work with the poor; what it is like for a middle-class family to "live with" the poor in what must be one of the very few experiments of its kind in the United States today to put doctors and homeless patients under the same roof; what it is like to walk *between* the worlds of the rich and the poor. This book is less about medicine than about race. My patients are overwhelmingly black because poverty in our nation's capital is primarily a black—although increasingly a Hispanic—phenomenon.[1] Everything a white doctor does—from choosing to practice in a black community in the first place to admitting patients to the large, mostly black community hospital rather than the small, wealthy, mostly white hospital across town to writing about his experiences for publication—brings the questions, confusions, and problems of race in America rushing to the fore.

This book is less about medicine than about culture. Great is the distance between a Yale-educated, third-generation white American and a poor, probably under-educated black person born in the rural South. From the entertainments we choose to the religious traditions we uphold, from our child-rearing practices to our beliefs about healing, from our family structures to our celebrations, my patients and I live in very different worlds. We struggle to share even a language.

This book is less about the medical treatment of esoteric diseases than about medical helplessness before the drugs of choice lodged so deeply in our society. When we think of inner-city addictions, most of us think of crack cocaine or heroin. In fact, the drug the reader will encounter most frequently in this book, the drug of most concern to me as a physician, the drug that—even in our neighborhood—does more damage than all the others combined, is alcohol.

This book is less about bold prescriptions for political or societal change than about what it's like to find oneself suddenly enmeshed in the crumbling relationship between government and the poor. It's about the grim consequences of two decades of governmental withdrawal and the deliberate underfunding of social agencies, about the helplessness of helpers running into the closed doors and cul-de-sacs of social policy. It is about the wholesale abandonment of the poor.

At its heart, then, this book is about the nature of poverty and its awful power to break the spirit. There are many poor people in the city of Washington who, with great courage, resist that power, get by more or less like middle-class people . . . only without money. Some of them are in this book. But because of the particular places at which I work and because of my focus on the homeless, this book is more about brokenness and failure, frustration and hopelessness than about successes and the hope they allow us.

I don't claim to have sorted out the complex linkages among race, poverty, and class in America any better than the many scholars and thinkers who have generated such a profusion of books on these subjects. In fact, although I've written many articles and stories about my work, although I've lectured widely to medical students and physicians about poverty medicine, I've found it difficult indeed to write this book. Because my form of medical practice tends to bring up virtually every large and confusing social issue and because life next to the poor revealed one contradiction after another in my own life, it was sometimes impossible to work out the nature of this "medical" book "about" a doctor. At several points I was simply unable to proceed for months on end, once for an entire year. My difficulties in writing only mirrored my problems as a poverty doctor. No matter how "simple" the medical problems I faced, I often found myself hopelessly lost in a forest of uncertainties.

What I can offer is primarily that I, a middle-class, white professional, have been *there* in that "other land"—a land that most of us see only when we stare into the face of a beggar insistently accosting us on the street or in brief, sanitized television reports that can be zapped off the screen—and that, with whatever hesitations, I want to be where I am.

I came to the inner city in part because I believed that poverty in our country was more a matter of *injustice* than of personal characteristics or bad luck, and because I believed in the possibility of justice. I came because I was aware, to some degree, of my privileged background, of the inherent power of a white male in our society. I came with the conviction that we who had grown up with education and opportunities had not so much deserved our affluence as inherited it and that the poor were—by virtue of their oppression—"deserving." I came, in other words, with hope: If poverty were the result of oppression, then even a small group of affluent people could make a difference by providing—through well-run service projects (subsidized housing, health centers, day-care and education institutions, job training, and other services)—the beginning of a way out. If injustice were the cause of poverty, then my presence as a health care provider would in some small way help my patients climb the "ladder" I knew was there.

I also came with a *desire* to help the poor, but (if I am honest) there was an element of obligation as well. For better or (usually) for worse I have operated much of my life out of a sense of "oughtness," and within my religious and cultural tradition there was certainly an ethical imperative to help the poor. Any relationship works both ways, however. What happens to a person when he—as an affluent, comfortable, well-intentioned physician—walks next to some of the barriers that ordinarily separate rich and poor? What happens when one who is wealthy° lives next to and works with people whose poverty is the result of the very structures that have brought him his wealth?

This, then, is a book about a journey, a journey that began both as a struggle against injustice on behalf of those abandoned by the rest of us and as a search for my own spiritual center. Though I knew the journey would be diffi-

° I use the term "wealthy" here and at other places in this book advisedly. Others would reserve the word for those rich enough to live off their assets alone or for those of inherited wealth or for those whose yearly income is over a certain figure or for those whose wealth brings them a certain level of political or social power. But wealth is simply an "abundance of valuable material possessions or resources." We affluent Americans (certainly those of us earning more than the median American income) who have money left after food, clothing, and shelter are paid for are—compared to the people of my neighborhood or certainly to the people of many developing countries—very wealthy.

cult, I thought that its goals and direction at least would be clear. I could not guess how deeply the struggle with the misery of the inner city would be mirrored in the chaos of my internal quest. My desire to understand the nature of that misery led me by turns to blame the rich, the poor, and myself for what I saw, and it led me also to a painful encounter with the limits of what I was capable of, and who I was.

My journey, of course, began long before I ever arrived in Washington, D.C. From 1975 until 1982, my family and I lived in the middle of a vast wilderness area in northeastern Minnesota, where I practiced family medicine. Marja, our three children (Laurel, Karin, and Kai), and I delighted in the stark beauty of the natural environment and in the intimacy of our small town. A rural community offers profound blessings to the doctor: I shared the joy of childbirth and the grief of illness or sudden death. I cherished the opportunity for trust between doctor and patient, and basked in the gratitude bestowed on the country doctor.

But the stress of rural medicine also took its toll. Living and working over one hundred miles from the nearest specialist, I needed to practice constantly at the limits of my competence—and frequently beyond: placing an emergency intracardiac pacemaker in a patient with a severe heart attack, although I hadn't done the procedure in years; performing a cesarean section on a friend, despite my inadequate surgical training; treating complex medical problems while repeatedly second-guessing myself about not referring the patient to a specialist's care in Duluth.

I found it difficult to be "the Doctor" in a small town where one could never be quite off-duty. When I was on call, I was not only the family doctor taking the late-afternoon telephone plea from the distraught mother, but also the emergency room physician evaluating the child's acute asthma attack later that evening. If necessary, I then became the pediatrician who admitted the child to the hospital a little before midnight and, sometimes, the house officer called down in the middle of the night to treat the worsening shortness of breath. If my pregnant patient came to afternoon office hours in labor, I could be sure to be up most of the night as I took turns being office doctor, telephone consultant, admitting physician, labor room nurse, delivering obstetrician, neonatal pediatrician, and finally honorary godfather. A few hours later I would be a pediatrician again, doing morning rounds on the newborn, and then general physician back in our clinic. It was wonderfully exhilarating . . . and unbearably exhausting.

It took me seven years to realize that the constant stress of my work no longer allowed me to receive the blessings of rural practice. I found myself frequently depressed, almost always anxious, sometimes terrified of going to work. I had chosen medicine in order to be of service to others, but I was unable to find the fulfillment I wanted from my life of service. I needed to leave.[2]

Our family moved for a year to Marja's home in Finland. There—amid natural beauty so similar to Minnesota's yet so far from the stress—I managed to recover my balance. Before leaving Minnesota, however, Marja and I had been introduced to Church of the Saviour, a small, ecumenical religious community in Washington, D.C., dedicated to working with poor people of the inner city. We thought of it often while we were away, and particularly of the efforts of one member.

In 1976 Janelle Goetcheus, a physician, and her husband Allen, a Methodist clergyman, while waiting for visas (which were ultimately not forthcoming) for traditional Christian missionary work in Southeast Asia, had visited Washington, where they witnessed the desperation of inner-city life and the absence of available medical care. The Goetcheuses were permanently detoured. Initially, Janelle worked in an emergency room and volunteered at various clinics, but soon she called together a group from Church of the Saviour to found Columbia Road Health Services, a small neighborhood clinic that burgeoned from a second-floor walk-up into the complete family-practice clinic that now sees over fifteen thousand patient visits a year, predominantly from the refugee Hispanic community. She also helped to establish Community of Hope Health Services, another family-practice clinic on nearby Belmont Street, and a third small clinic at SOME (So Others May Eat), a soup kitchen sponsored by the Catholic Church. Although sponsored by separate organizations, the three clinics functioned as a loosely knit group practice providing health services to the poor. In early 1983 I accepted the invitation to join her in her work.

Even after a year's rest and contemplation, my motivation in coming to Washington was not clear to me. I experienced a vague sense that my own fulfillment was to be found in a life among the poor, but I was not sure whether I felt that way or merely wanted to feel that way, whether my motivation was simply an internalization of certain biblical texts and childhood messages or whether it was really my own belief. I certainly couldn't talk about what I was doing without becoming quickly confused, all the more so since a move from an idyllic wilderness area to inner-city Washington hardly made sense: If I had not been able to tolerate practice in a small, supportive town, how was I to survive the inner city?

In some ways, however, practice in the city actually proved easier. My partners and I soon realized that what the city's poor really needed was *access* to the health care system, frontline doctors offering primary care who could help them connect with the wider system. With an abundance of specialists around, I no longer delivered babies, set fractures, or took care of complicated medical problems. When patients called in the middle of the night, I remained a family doctor and referred them to an emergency room for evaluation. I soon stopped hospital practice and the acute care of seriously ill people altogether.

Not only did the changes in my role give me some hope of surviving the stress, but I also entered into a *community* of persons all engaged in similar work, and we were remarkably supportive of one another. For all its drawbacks,

it seemed that poverty medicine might suit me better than
any "normal" practice.

Despite my eagerness, however, there was no way to prepare myself to face the unraveling of the social fabric, the
larger loss of community that was the truth of inner-city
Washington. I was initially shocked and angry at a system
that had abandoned those least able to help themselves.
There was no housing; medical care was inaccessible; public education was a disaster; jobs with living wages were
unavailable. Most of my new patients had the same kinds
of medical illnesses I had tended in Minnesota, but they
also suffered from a kind of neglect I had not imagined
possible.

That shock, though, I could at least see coming. What
caught me completely off guard was my patients' internalization of their abandonment. Children who had not been
adequately loved now saw themselves as unlovable; young
people who had been inadequately trusted could now trust
no one; adults who had been pushed down too many times
now saw failure as inevitable; addicts for whom no treatment was offered had now—for practical purposes—given
up on the possibility of a meaningful life. I was not prepared for the hostility, the seeming ingratitude, the noncompliance, the irrationality that is so much a part of the
inner-city reality.

This was a journey into a strange and threatening world.

There are a variety of obstacles any middle-class reader is
likely to face in accompanying me on this journey. Not the
least, for some readers, will be its religious aspect. I am the
son of a clergyman, reared in a mainline Protestant church.
Although as a young adult I left the church for over fifteen
years, I always felt a vocation to serve others. The decision
to enter the inner city was born of a conscious desire to
move into a closer relationship with God. When Marja and I
joined Janelle Goetcheus, we did so as much for the opportunity to live and work within a Christian spiritual community as for the chance to practice a certain kind of medicine.

Some readers, coming across names like "Christ House" or "Samaritan Inn," may feel imposed upon, even though ours is an ecumenical church community that emphasizes spiritual growth and acts of mercy and advocacy rather than doctrine or theological correctness. Isn't it enough, some readers may nonetheless feel, to bring oneself to a book on homelessness and poverty—a book that has every possibility of being amply guilt-inducing—without having to deal with the self-righteousness of the church? I often discover such wariness when I talk to medical audiences about poverty medicine. For some, the very existence of a religious mission at the core of my practice is grounds for dismissal: of me, of poverty medicine, of the homeless, of any connection between the middle class and the poor. For others, the spiritual dimension to our doctoring can evoke images of paternalistic missionary work, of the white man and his culture ultimately disempowering poor people of color by "serving" them. If this were the "religion" hawked in this book, I would have none of it either.

A reader who does not personally experience religion as a source of strength may be tempted to dismiss the "religiously motivated" as saints or lunatics (the distinction is not always obvious to the uninitiated) whose purposes and life experiences have little to do with one's own. Medical students with whom I talk sometimes say, "I can see how *you* might survive in the inner city, with your Christian community and your faith in God and God's healing, but what about me? I have no religious faith and no community. How is your experience in any way relevant to mine?"

I usually answer that *each* of us is on a spiritual journey, articulated or not, and our deepest beliefs invariably shape who we are. My religious beliefs do inform my decisions to live and practice in Washington's inner city, but that makes me little different from any other person trying consciously and reflectively to live according to his or her convictions. God, according to all religious traditions, lives within each of us. Any person trying to live by attending to that "deep stillness within"—whether expressed in Christian, Jewish,

Islamic, Buddhist, Native American, or absolutely secular
language—should find him- or herself at home with the
spirituality (and, I hope, with the language) in this book.
More practically, if one dismisses spiritual (or even ex-
plicitly religious) motivation for medical work with the
inner-city poor—in Washington, at least—there's not much
left to talk about in the 1990s except the leaching of all
care from the ever-growing worlds of poverty and homelessness. In the 1980s, as government money was withdrawn from the ghettos, as private investment never
entered, as community organizing petered out, as a few private practitioners struggled (too often unsuccessfully) to
make ends meet while caring for the indigent, often all that
was left were church groups and other parareligious organizations trying against overwhelming odds to address even
the barest, most basic needs of the poor.

My own hope is that even those who find religious labels
and beliefs embarrassing or irrelevant will find something
for themselves here. "Religious" or not, conscious of it or
not, safely ensconced in the suburbs or not, each of us is in-
extricably bound to—indeed, tangled up with—the pain of
the poor. My hope is to reveal some of those bonds, to acknowledge our common community.

One last concern: It is dangerous, and ultimately mislead-
ing, to speak—as I frequently do in the pages to follow—of
"the poor," for this implies a homogeneity that does not exist. Poor people are not an indistinguishable mass, and the
causes of poverty are multiple.

I have, in fact, only a single fear in offering this book,
but that fear almost keeps me from publishing. It would be
easy for the reader to infer from many of the specific poor
or homeless people I write about that virtually all inner-city
people are addicted, mentally ill, incompetent, or otherwise
severely damaged. It is possible that a superficial acquain-
tance with the people I introduce here will only reinforce
stereotypes and prejudices about the poor as lazy, hostile,
ungrateful, inadequate. If this book results in such an exten-

sion of our already sizable hatred for the poor, I will have contributed to the problem rather than to its solution. Like any other group of people, my patients vary enormously in talent and ability, health and intelligence. But the nature of my work as an inner-city physician is to attend to those particular urban poor people who are doing the least well. The reader will not meet too many inspiring people in this book, not because there are no such individuals in my practice but because it is the others who have had such a profound impact on my life. There are obviously many poor people—and many in my practice—who need little else but justice: a temporary place to stay, a decent education, a chance to work, access to health care, affordable housing. But there are also multitudes so broken that such improvements will have little overall effect on their lives. The "liberal" inclination to see in economic and political oppression the causes of poverty must not blind us to the fact that an unjust society produces a kind of brokenness that cannot always be redressed simply by removing the injustice.

All of the stories in this book are stories of real people. Because the writing often occurred years after the events, certain details and dialogues may not be exact, although I have done my best to make them so. With the exception of colleagues and some public officials, however, the names of those who appear here have been changed and details of their stories have frequently been intentionally altered, sometimes enough to make individuals unrecognizable even to themselves. Where this was not possible, I have shared the stories with those involved and they have not only given me permission to tell their stories but have actively encouraged me to do so. To them I am grateful.

Chapter 2

First Days

In September 1983, Marja and I moved to the inner city of Washington, D.C., with our three children—Laurel, who was twelve years old; Karin, who was about to turn nine; and Kai, who was four. We rented the top two floors of a brick, three-story row house in the rapidly changing Mount Pleasant neighborhood, three miles due north from the White House. The neighborhoods on each side of us could not have been more different. Two blocks to the east lay one of Washington's mini-ghettos, where, in the heat and mugginess of those September evenings, adults still congregated on the steps of the run-down apartment buildings, the sidewalks, and the other open spaces while children played in the streets and alleys. A constant stream of cars moved slowly through the street, for an active drug market flourished exactly where the young children played, with older children often acting as "runners" for only slightly older sellers. Two blocks to the west of us were old, well-kept row houses in a quiet, middle-class, racially integrated neighborhood bordering on the wide swath of Rock Creek Park, which swept across our northern border. Two blocks to the south was a slightly shabby business strip, an area quickly becoming the center of a large community of Salvadoran refugees.

Driving to Community of Hope Health Services for my first day of work, I was struck by the ever-shifting patchwork of people and languages, races and cultures, affluence and poverty that made up my new community. As Janelle and I left her comfortably air-conditioned apartment in the Adams-Morgan neighborhood just south of Mount Pleasant for the Health Services on Belmont Street less than a mile away, I watched the neighborhood change with every block. Some fine old apartment buildings like that of the Goetcheuses remained from a time thirty years earlier when the whole neighborhood had been well-to-do and predominantly white. The single-family row houses on the next blocks were still occupied by the middle-class families— black and white—that had owned them for a generation. The streets were lined with large shade trees, a few children played on the sidewalks, and people on stoops chatted with neighbors. Gentrification was beginning, Janelle told me; young professionals, white and black, were buying homes and apartments in the area at ever-increasing prices.

As we crossed Columbia Road, we were quite suddenly out of the residential neighborhood. This was another aspect of the city. Paper and bottles were strewn everywhere. A young woman waiting to cross the street in front of us casually dropped an empty potato chip bag on the street within twenty feet of a trash can; boys smashed a soda bottle on the curbstone. Men and women rushed by, oblivious. Even in the morning heat of over ninety degrees, the sidewalks were busy. Four white men who—in their suits and ties—looked to be in their early thirties emerged together from a Mexican restaurant and walked briskly by a black homeless man dozing on his milk crate, his hat upside down on the sidewalk in front of him. A group of black children ran up the street through knots of Hispanic men. Latin music blasted from a hidden boom box.

Barely a block later, we were back in a residential, though not affluent, area. We passed H. D. Cook Elementary School, an old-fashioned, rectangular brick building in back of which lay a grim asphalt playground. Across the street, near abandoned apartment buildings, separate groups of young black and Hispanic men clustered, eyeing one another warily. Janelle pointed out the Ritz and the Mozart, once-elegant apartment buildings that—during the sixties and early seventies—had become dilapidated tenements until purchased and renovated as low-cost housing by small "mission groups" from Church of the Saviour. Spilling out of the nondescript red-brick apartment buildings were children of all ages. On the corner a group of young men waited. Once again, paper litter blew everywhere and bottles lay broken on both street and sidewalk.

Another block and the neighborhood was cleaner, newer: a ten-story high-rise offered housing for students from Howard University. A large air-conditioned bus waited out front to shuttle the students to and from the campus, ten blocks away. Across the street was Malcolm X Park.

Although in Washington there are few rigid geographical dividing lines separating the well-off from the poor, Malcolm X Park, sitting atop Meridian Hill, marks a very real border. It is a lovely place to walk in daylight, with an ornate garden, winding paths, a spectacular cascading waterfall, and beautiful reflecting pools that invite meditation. Groups of either African or Hispanic immigrants (but never mixed groups) seem always to have a soccer game in progress. At night, according to local residents, the park belongs to a different element of the city: The drug sellers move in from Chapin Street, two blocks to the east, and young girls trade sex for crack among the bushes and in dark corners. But during the day, one feels very much a part of a comfortable, affluent culture in the nation's capital.

A few blocks later, on Fourteenth Street, it was hard to believe we were in the same city. Lots lay vacant; storefronts were boarded up. Scores of people milled around in one of the largest open-air drug markets in the city; police waited in cars on the corner, apparently unable to do anything. Behind a complex of three large, run-down apartment buildings stood another: a burned-out reminder of the riots that followed Martin Luther King's assassination. One block farther, we turned onto Belmont Street, a two-way street that officially became one-way at sunset in order to prevent suburban cars from driving back and forth, cruising for drugs. (As far as I could tell, no one ever paid much attention to the prohibition.) ˎ

We parked near the corner, the spot where the first fires of the 1968 riots were reportedly set. The gutted shells of the buildings had been razed years ago, and now only the empty lots remained, barren markers of the area's desolation, stark illustrations of how little help or money has entered such communities since. Just up the hill was the Pitts Hotel, once a symbol of black elegance, home to visiting entertainers and other important guests, but now a city shelter where—I was to learn later—a wealthy black businessman charged the city nearly $2,500 a month to shelter and feed *each* of fifty-two homeless families.

As we made our way up the block, a stream of people came toward us—homeless families, Janelle told me, from other shelters in the city. The Pitts, the city's first shelter for homeless families, still remained the only source of meals and social services even though growing numbers of families were now being housed "temporarily" at run-down motels around the city. These families now had to take crosstown buses three times a day from their scattered motels just to get meals. Women, their children in tow, were walking down to the bus stop on the corner: on their way to look for jobs, as the public assistance program required them to do every day.

In the middle of the block stood Community of Hope; it looked little different from the other four-story brick tenements I'd seen on my drive over. In front was a small yard worn to rock-hard yellow dirt. Numerous attempts to create something green on the space finally ended several years later with brick being laid across the entire surface. An alley—strewn with trash—ran up the side and across the back of the building. The heat was stultifying. People clustered in the shade, talking or just looking; children seemed to appear from anywhere and disappear just as quickly.

Janelle and I climbed the steps into the building, entering a long, dimly lit hallway. In 1976 Tom Nees, pastor of the affluent, predominantly white Church of the Nazarene on upper Sixteenth Street, and a small group from his middle-class congregation purchased the boarded-up tenement next to the empty lots. It had long been abandoned; its only residents were eighteen-year-old Rita Branham and her children, squatting there without heat, water, or electricity. Nees and his group began transforming the building into a usable structure, starting with the apartment in which Rita and her children were staying. They also founded in the building a small Church of the Nazarene mission congregation that, within a few years, grew into an active independent church with a broad range of services. Tom Nees's sister, Lois Wagner, moved with her family from Los Angeles to open a medical clinic there, and Janelle began her doctoring. A children's program was developed—babysitting for young children, tutoring for school-age children, summer camp programs, and special clubs. The apartments in Community of Hope were renovated and a contract signed with the city to begin the Families-in-Transition program (FIT): Fifteen formerly homeless families moved in and, over the course of the three to six months that they were allowed to stay, received medical attention, social services, and assistance in locating permanent housing. As each family moved out into its own apartment, a new family from the city shelter system moved in. Later on, a jobs-readiness training program was developed. Although not formally part of Community of Hope, a group of young lawyers established an office and practice in the building as well, providing full-time, affordable legal help to the residents of the building and other neighbors. Community of Hope had become a full-fledged social service agency. Rita Branham had stayed on, working in various capacities at Community of Hope and eventually becoming administrative director for the entire organization.

Janelle and I walked down the long hallway and opened the wooden door into the clinic. An electric fan on the receptionist's desk did little to lighten the heavy air. The long, narrow waiting room was packed: Two small children sat coloring at a small table; next to them an unshaven older man in a dark, stained suit simply stared. A young woman near the reception desk in the middle of the room was scolding a child in a dialect so difficult to understand I could barely recognize it as English; two teenagers lounged along the wall to our right; and a heavyset, middle-aged woman, the only white person in the room, nodded in the corner behind us. As we entered, the room became suddenly quiet. People looked at us, sat up straighter, and drew their feet in so we could pass through the waiting room.

There was nothing ornate about the clinic. It was clean, bright, and cheery, but it was clear that little money had been spent on decoration. The blue rug was frayed, and the cream-colored, bare plaster walls—while newly painted—did not hide their long history. Water marks from leaks on the second floor stained the ceiling at irregular intervals. Portraits of neighborhood people by Tom's wife, Pat Nees, hung on the walls.

Apparently alerted by the receptionist, a petite, attractive, middle-aged woman with short, prematurely white hair hurried in through a side door. I guessed her to be the director, Lois Wagner. "You must be Dr. Hilfiker," she said to me and turned immediately to Janelle. "You're just in time. Suggs is having another seizure." She led us back through the same side door, down another dark hallway, and into a large room appointed—except for a desk covered with papers in one corner—like a living room. Suggs, a tall, gaunt black man, lay stretched out on the old couch, his eyes closed, snoring spasmodically, a thin stream of spittle drooling from the corner of his mouth. "I guess he's all right," Lois said. "He seems to know when he's going to have one. He said he stopped drinking yesterday and hasn't taken his Dilantin in several weeks. Then he started shaking and went into a full-blown seizure. Just like two months ago."

Janelle bent over him, felt his pulse, touched his forehead. "His blood pressure was okay when I took it," said Lois.

Janelle straightened up. "I guess there's not much to do. Call the ambulance, I suppose, so he can be watched for a day or two in the hospital while they get his Dilantin regulated." All three of us stood looking down at Suggs, perhaps embarrassed at our helplessness. I had literally done nothing, but my shirt was soaked with sweat. Lois looked at me and laughed. "Welcome to Washington! Come on over to the lab. There's an air conditioner we huddle around when it gets like this." She led me back through the throng in the waiting room and into a tiny room, its shelves lined with prescription medication hustled from pharmaceutical company representatives and stocked with rudimentary medical testing equipment. The temperature dropped into the almost-comfortable range. Behind a refrigerator, an air conditioner labored noisily in the window at the far end of the room.

Janelle left to see her first patient, and Lois was temporarily called out to the desk. I found myself alone in the small room with a few moments to think. The chaos of the city, Suggs and his seizure, a waiting room full of strange patients; this was probably going to be "normal," but it seemed suddenly overwhelming. I had had a difficult time in a relatively protected and peaceful environment in Minnesota. How would I survive this?

Soon Lois returned to show me through the rest of the clinic. It was a sprawling maze of small rooms and narrow hallways that had obviously been built piecemeal, moving some walls here, knocking out others there. Seven different doors and passageways opened off the central waiting room, leading into various rooms and hallways from which one then entered exam rooms, counseling offices, a business office, storage rooms, and restrooms. A distant corner had been made into a small kitchen. One restroom could be reached only by walking through a tiny office sometimes used for counseling.

It seemed a long time before I heard the wail of the ambulance. I returned to the crowded waiting room just in time to see three fully equipped, uniformed paramedics walk into the room. "Somebody's havin' a seizure?" the man in front asked. He seemed bored . . . or was he simply resentful at our call? I led them into Lois's room. Suggs stood up, wobbling, as we entered. "I'm all right," he said, his eyes still glazed. "I'm all right." He stumbled backward against the table.

"This the guy?" asked the first man, taking out a blood pressure cuff and sitting Suggs back on the couch.

Suggs stood up again, wobbling. He looked down at his feet. "I'll be all right," he said to Lois as she came in. "It was just a little one. Won't do no good to go over to Howard. I just gotta take my medicine."

The paramedic drew back. "We can't force you to go, you know."

Lois interrupted. "He didn't say he didn't want to go." She turned to Suggs. "Dr. Goetcheus thinks you should go to the hospital, Suggs. Why don't you go on over just to get checked out?"

Suggs looked up at the paramedic and, again, down at his feet. "No, I don't think I should go," he mumbled, and staggered out to sit in the waiting room. While the paramedics lingered impatiently, Lois tried to convince Suggs to go, but his mind was made up. The paramedic gave Suggs a form to sign, to document that he was refusing ambulance attention. When I checked in a little later, Suggs was no longer there.

I did not have any responsibility in any of this, but I could feel my frustration rising. Here was a man with a significant set of medical problems, which in Minnesota would have required at least further testing and probably admission to the hospital; but here the paramedics seemed only too willing to let him stay on the streets, and he himself, for whatever reason, did not protest. Indeed, he seemed reluctant to accept further care.

If I felt overwhelmed and confused by my first days in Washington, I was not alone. Don Martin, a family physician ten years older than I who had left his private practice of twenty years to join Janelle the same week I did, shared my sense of helplessness. Don worked at another of the clinics Janelle had begun, Columbia Road Health Services, which provided care primarily to Central American refugees. Don didn't speak Spanish and therefore worked with a translator, most frequently Gloria Gomez, a young nurse from Uruguay. Translation from one language to the other, however, was only the first and probably the easiest obstacle to understanding.

Typical for Don and Gloria was their experience with Maria Elena Florez, a young Salvadoran mother. When Don and Gloria interviewed her, she complained of disabling headaches. On further interview and examination Don could find no physical cause for her symptoms and so made a diagnosis of tension headaches, not unusual considering the stress under which refugees like Maria Elena lived. Gloria then remained in the room to give the patient a few simple instructions on the treatment of her headaches, while Don returned to his office cubicle to dictate his chart note, write a prescription for a mild pain reliever for Maria Elena, and answer a telephone call from another patient. Don soon finished his phone call, but Gloria—still in the exam room with Maria Elena—was not available to translate for the next patient, who also spoke only Spanish. Needing to move on if he was to see all his patients that morning, Don arranged to examine someone else from the waiting room who spoke passable English. After he was finished, Gloria had still not returned. Don finally interrupted Gloria, only to find both her and Maria Elena in tears.

Maria Elena and her husband had fled their home in war-torn El Salvador, leaving their five young children in the care of an aunt. For weeks now they had had no news of their children. An "illegal alien" in a foreign land whose language she did not understand, Maria Elena was always fearful of deportation. Her husband—under the same pressures—had just recently been fired from his job as a waiter because someone had reported his employer to the Immigration and Naturalization Service; he had also started drinking and was beating her regularly. And now, the hospital where she had just given birth to her daughter was dunning her on account of bills she could not pay. Although her newborn—an American citizen by birth—was technically eligible for Medicaid, Maria Elena herself qualified for no assistance at all. Furthermore, she was afraid to apply for her daughter's Medicaid, for fear of being reported to Immigration.

Gloria could translate for Don, but how could either of them offer anything except their presence to this young woman? When Maria Elena returned a week later, tearfully reporting that the prescribed heat and massage to her neck had done nothing for her headaches and the pills were upsetting her stomach, how were they to respond? Problems that bore a superficial similarity to ones Don had treated for twenty years in private practice were, on further examination, infinitely more complex.

Don and I would see many patients like Suggs and Maria Elena as the weeks went on. And many of the things that initially disturbed us began to seem familiar, even normal. We got used to the ways of the office. It no longer seemed odd that the receptionist had to write down a patient's address and phone number at every visit, for phones are disconnected regularly in this community and addresses are fluid. It no longer seemed unusual that Lois had to conduct patient-intake interviews behind a file cabinet in the waiting room. I got used to changing a person's blood pressure medication every few months, not because of any problem with the initial medication but because we had run out of free samples. Sometimes it even seemed that we were little different from any other doctor's office; we were, after all, still performing the basic functions—examining patients, making diagnoses, prescribing medications. But there was always something unexpected, a reminder of where we were.

Just now the patient is Monica Jackson, a thin, thirty-year-old black woman who is distraught. I hear her talking loudly at Lois during check-in: "Where is he? I gotta see him right away. How long is it gonna be?" She gets up and paces around the waiting room, staying close to the reception desk, avoiding the door to the hallway. Lois finally brings her into the exam room. "Doc, you gotta help me. I got somethin' stuck down there, an' I can't get it out. You gotta get it out right away. I tried but I couldn't reach in far enough." She is nervous; her hands move quickly. Intermittently, the muscles under her right eyebrow twitch as if she were winking at me. "You've got something stuck in your vagina?" I ask. "What is it?" She looks down, wringing her hands. She gives no answer. Not wanting to embarrass her, I don't press; I've been in this position before, usually finding an old tampon or perhaps a condom lodged high in the vagina. "Take off your bottoms and put this sheet over your lap," I say. "I'll be in with the nurse in a minute to take a look."

On pelvic examination it is not difficult to find what I'm looking for. At first it looks like the condom I expect, a small wad of plastic that I grab easily with a long-handled ring forceps and remove. It's not a condom, however, but a good-sized plastic bag. And the bag contains white powder. I look over at the nurse, tell Monica to get dressed, and leave the room.

I am confused. The powder is obviously some drug— probably heroin, although I can't, myself, tell it from any other—but what is it doing *there*? And what am I supposed to do now? Fortunately, there are lawyers at the other end of the building. I call down to ask for advice. After some consultation, I am informed that since the drug is now in my possession, I am legally guilty of heroin *distribution* if I do anything but give it to the police. I could be prosecuted, the lawyer reminds me.

I return to the exam room without the heroin. Monica is dressed, sitting nervously in the corner. "Ms. Jackson, I don't know how or why that package got there, but I can't give it back to you. Once it comes into my hands, I can't give it back to you without breaking the law myself. I'm going to have to turn it over to the police."

Her face drains and her mouth falls open. A look of absolute terror comes into her eyes. For a moment she is speechless, then tears flow, and the words pour out. "You gotta give it back, Doc. I was just holdin' it and they was gonna give me a piece. I can't pay for all that. They'll kill me if I don't give it back. They'll think I took it and sold it or used it. My life won't be worth nothin'. You don't know those people. They'd just as soon shoot you as look at you, and they ain't gonna let nobody get away with not givin' them their shit back." She looks at me wildly. "You gotta give it back."

I try to look at her levelly. "I'm sorry, but it would be against the law. Once I take it out, I become liable for it. I can't give it back."

"Why didn't you tell me that? I should've never come in here. Doc, they're gonna kill me, you know that?" Tears are streaming down her face. "I should never have come here." She slides from the chair and actually kneels before me, grabbing my hands. "You gotta give it back to me. You don't know those people."

I don't know what to do. I extricate my hands from hers, stand up, call in the nurse to stay with her, and walk into the medication room where it will at least be cool. My shirt is soaking wet. In desperation, I finally phone Janelle for advice. "I guess it wouldn't have occurred to me to ask a legal opinion," she finally says. "I would have just assumed I'd have to give it back to her."

"Well, now you have the legal opinion," I say. "What would you do now?"

Her normally soft voice trails off. "That's a hard one. That's a hard one."

I hang up the phone, put the package in my pocket, walk back into the exam room, and ask the nurse to leave us alone. I'm not sure what I'm doing, and I don't want anyone else to be responsible for my decision. Without saying a word, I give the packet to Monica. She looks at me with disbelieving eyes, then jumps up and hugs me awkwardly. The tears continue to pour down. She sits back down and looks at me. "I gotta stop this, y'know." For the first time I notice the needle tracks on her forearms. "I been shootin' this shit for twelve years. I gotta stop it."

"We might be able to arrange treatment for you, Monica. Providence Hospital would probably take you in for a monthlong treatment program. You could kick it if you wanted to."

She nods and looks down. "I know," she says quietly. Then her eyes brighten. "I gotta take care of this. Then I'll be back. Maybe you can find somethin' for me. I'll be back this afternoon right away. Or maybe tomorrow." She looks me in the eyes. "I promise."

It's the last I ever see of her.

Occasionally an element of the truly bizarre entered into my encounters, an image that would etch itself indelibly in my memory and a reminder that this would never become familiar territory.

I first read about Joanne Torson just after my arrival at Community of Hope; she was the subject of a *Washington Post* article on drug traffic in the city. Thirty-seven, she was the proprietress of an "oil joint," an apartment where junkies could come with their heroin and pay her five dollars (or a portion of their supply) to have her inject it for them. For the many whose previous injections had destroyed the superficial veins in their arms and legs, Joanne would inject directly into one of the large blood vessels in the neck. This was not, the columnist wrote, so unusual. What *was* unusual was the fact that Joanne had only one arm! Repeated injections of heroin in the other arm had led to "burns" (open sores on the skin), to infection, and finally to amputation. "One-Hand Joanne" was her moniker. As a physician used to drawing blood, I had a hard time believing anyone could do it one-handed, but Joanne's skill was legendary in Washington's intravenous-drug-using community.

The official response to the *Post* article came several days later, when Joanne was arrested and then admitted to D.C. General Hospital for detoxification. A week later, however, she was discharged from the hospital to the jail, where she was promptly released on a ten-dollar bond. Since she lived not far from Community of Hope and Tom Nees had contacted her during her detox, she called him from the jail, and he brought her to his office upstairs. Tom suggested I come up to get acquainted with Joanne and see if I could be of help in getting her into a drug treatment program.

As I walked into his spacious, well-lighted office on the second floor, I was momentarily taken aback. Somehow I had expected a heavyset, scowling, angry woman, turning a bitter face to the world. Instead, a wisp of a woman sat near the window in a simple patterned cotton dress, eating carry-out Chinese from a nearby storefront. Bathed in natural light, her face seemed decidedly childlike as she turned toward me. She smiled and said she was pleased to meet me. It was then I noticed that not only was her left arm missing, but her right leg had also been amputated just below the hip. Her remaining arm was grotesquely swollen, and I could see blood-tinged serum oozing through the thin bandages from the "burns" on that arm, too. It did not take an expert to predict that—unless she stopped injecting drugs, had the best medical care, and was very lucky besides—gangrene and amputation of that arm, too, would not be far in the future.

The immediate problem was what to do next. Joanne had just been discharged from D.C. General with no medications or follow-up. While she was in the hospital, her doctors had given her forty milligrams of methadone daily to detoxify her from the heroin, but they had made no provision for her to continue receiving it once out of the hospital. I knew that as a community physician I would not be able to write her a prescription for methadone; in the United States, it is one of the very few legal drugs prescribed only from within a hospital or specified drug treatment center. Even with my then-limited experience, I also knew that it would take at least four weeks to enroll her at Karrick Hall, the city's twenty-eight-day inpatient alcohol treatment unit available to those without money, and five or six weeks to enroll her in the city's outpatient methadone program. While waiting, she was—supposedly—to stay free of the heroin to which she had been continuously addicted for seventeen years. Joanne was very clear: "If they don't give me somethin', I can tell you I'll be on the street tonight. They take me off the meth and don't give me nothin' else, no way I can stay clean. No way I can do it on my own. I tried before, and I was right back out there. Won't be no different this time."

"What did the doctors say when they discharged you?" I asked.

"Oh, they said not to worry about it; I'd get the medicines I needed. They didn't give me bandages for these burns either."

What were the hospital physicians thinking of? I called D.C. General to try to find out. I talked with a resident physician-in-training, who had taken care of Joanne and discharged her from the hospital. Joanne, he said, had been under arrest while in the hospital and had been discharged directly to the jail. It was against hospital regulations to give *any* medications or prescriptions to patients who were discharged to the jail. Once incarcerated, she would get her methadone and other medicines, he told me, directly from the prison system.

But as soon as Joanne arrived at D.C. Jail (on the same physical campus as the hospital), she was, as is customary for a nonviolent drug offender, freed on the ten-dollar bond she'd mentioned to me. That meant, naturally, that it was no longer the jail's responsibility to find her the medications she needed. It was a scenario straight from *Catch-22*. The resident, undoubtedly struggling hard enough to learn the intricacies of *scientific* medicine, was simply unaware that as a D.C. General Hospital physician he could have discharged Joanne directly into the public outpatient methadone program; nor did he realize that community physicians would have to wait weeks to get her into such a program once she had been discharged. Tom was in the process of arranging transportation to Virginia, where Joanne's daughter lived. I wrote out prescriptions for medications that might ease, if only slightly, the effects of withdrawal. The next morning our social worker would try to get Joanne back on Medicaid and, once that came through, admitted to a private in-hospital detoxification program. Sometime in the future, possibly, we could attend to the chronic ulcers on her limbs, which would entail a difficult set of medical problems. But it was clear that, without somebody doing something above and beyond the ordinary routines *today*, Joanne would be back on heroin in the morning.

Joanne did get into Karrick Hall, but only because of a fortuitous combination of fate and politics. The next day, while at a social function, Tom mentioned Joanne's situation privately to the D.C. commissioner of health. Recognizing the potential public embarrassment to the city if the subject of the recent newspaper article were unable to get treatment, the commissioner (according to Tom) literally ran to the phone to bypass the system and make arrangements for Joanne's admission.

After discharge from Karrick Hall, Joanne never returned to the clinic, despite our invitation. I saw her only one other time, after a surgeon had suggested skin grafts for the worst of her ulcers. Prior to the scheduled surgery, Joanne needed blood drawn for tests, but she couldn't get to the hospital easily, and her children had called the clinic to ask if someone could come over to the house to draw blood. I volunteered, mostly because I was interested in seeing how and where she lived.

Joanne's children, two meticulously groomed young people in their late teens or early twenties, met me at the door. Both, I learned later, had finished school, had good jobs, and had moved to the suburbs. I couldn't imagine how they had escaped their mother's chaos to lead such apparently successful lives. Joanne lay on an old sofa in the living room. Her physical condition was even worse than I anticipated. A putrid odor filled the room . . . pus from an infection on the skin, I guessed. Under her nightgown, Joanne's body was clearly emaciated. I had not really appreciated the extent of her skin ulcers when I saw her in Tom's office. Not only were her remaining arm and leg covered with sores (a few coalesced into open wounds half a foot in diameter), there were even ulcers on the stumps of her amputated arm and leg. Many of the ulcers were filled with the white-gray pus I smelled.

She was unwilling to come to the office or consider immediate hospitalization for her infections, but she did want her blood drawn. After four tries, though, I gave up: She simply had no superficial veins that I could find, and here in her house, I didn't have the equipment for, nor did I want to attempt, the more dangerous arterial puncture. In parting I asked if she was still clean, and she nodded and smiled, almost sweetly. On my way out, however, her children were quick to tell me that she was using again. They didn't know what to do.

I didn't, either.

My introduction to the city had begun.

Chapter 3

WAR STORIES

I was not completely naïve about the realities of urban America, even in rural Minnesota. When I was very young, my family lived in a black St. Louis ghetto, where my father was the director of a settlement house. After college and during medical school, I lived for periods of time in the inner cities of New Haven, Connecticut, and St. Paul, Minnesota. I knew from personal observation, as well as my studies, that our cities were in deep trouble. I had read about the lack of housing and jobs and heard stories of the lack of access to adequate medical care. I had some sense—intellectually, at least—of the damage to people's lives involved. What I was not prepared for during those first months in Washington, however, was the *injustice*; how the myriad forms of poverty, woven together, formed a web from which escape—even with superhuman effort— was almost impossible.

My naïveté lay perhaps in my hope. I believed that if we in Church of the Saviour could offer good medical care to some few poor people in the inner city at a reasonable cost, this might serve as a model for others, perhaps even for governmental programs. If we could demonstrate to other physicians and medical professionals that our practice brought the personal fulfillment that most medical people had entered their profession to find, it might encourage others to build similar nonprofit structures. Was it not at least possible for us to call the medical profession back to its traditional responsibility to the poor? If we, through our speeches and writings, told the story of inner-city pain to a broad enough audience, it might turn individual compassion into social compassion, which would then translate into political action. Equal opportunity was a fundamental American promise: Surely, then, it was possible to offer the citizens of the American inner city at least basic medical care!

I was not dissuaded from my hopefulness in the early days of practice. Despite my initial experiences with patients like John Turnell, Suggs, and Monica Jackson, the medical problems my inner-city patients brought to the office seemed, on the whole, not so different from those I'd taken care of in rural Minnesota. Things were, perhaps, not as bad as I'd thought. Certainly there was pain and suffering here, but as a rural physician I had become familiar enough with tragedy. Addictions, abandonment, despair, physical deformity, severe illness, death are hardly confined to the ghetto. A primary-care doctor anywhere becomes accustomed to working with patients who hold little hope for their future.

Of course, Washington's multicultural patient population did not look like my Minnesota Scandinavians, and they certainly spoke with new accents. From the beginning I recognized there were cultural barriers here that I might never cross. I knew I might never know this new community as intimately as I had known my community in Minnesota. Even so, my doctoring in the inner city was, from a certain perspective, remarkably similar to my previous work. My patients still brought me their high blood pressure, their diabetes, their swollen joints; they still suffered from loneliness and depression; they still struggled with alcohol or other substances; they still came to the office, it seemed to me, more for support and reassurance than for a cure.

Nor did my own daily rhythm change significantly. I came from the comfort of my own home to an office. I talked with and examined patients in the privacy and insularity of the exam room. I made essentially the same medical decisions, recommended most of the same treatments I had as a country doctor. The clinic in Washington was perhaps more makeshift than the one in Minnesota, the exam room door flimsier (allowing perhaps a bit more noise from the hallway); nevertheless, once I closed that door, the chaos I sensed "out there" seemed more distant, and I could imagine—without too much stretching—that I was just like any other doctor with his patient. But there would be times when not even the exam room door would protect me.

Some months after I had begun working in Washington, Sister Lenora Benda called me from the large downtown shelter operated by the Community for Creative Non-Violence. Lenora had begun her career as a nurse practitioner in the refugee camps of Thailand and had next chosen to work among the "refugees" of our own culture. She had recently begun visiting the city shelters as part of a new program to bring health care to the homeless.

Could I "squeeze in" one of her patients? The lab had just reported back results on Louise Flowers, who appeared to be having some thyroid trouble; Lenora wanted me to evaluate her.

My 11:30 patient had just canceled—actually calling ahead to tell us—so I was open to Lenora's request. In my Minnesota practice, I had always flinched when someone suggested squeezing in another patient. I had never figured out how to "squeeze" my response to the needs of one person in order to accommodate the needs of another. So in Minnesota the phrase usually meant my staying late and ignoring some other, perhaps family, responsibility or personal desire. The alternative—doing the squeezing by cutting patients off before they were really finished—was for me the more painful.

One of the paradoxical blessings of my work at Community of Hope, however, was that almost half my patients didn't show up for their appointments, so I usually had time for the unexpected. "Walk-ins" could most likely be seen even without appointment. Although our schedule book was full at the beginning of any given day, I frequently saw more walk-ins than scheduled patients. I had become more relaxed about "squeezing" someone in.

"Why don't you send her over about eleven o'clock, Lenora? Have her bring copies of the lab work with her." I return to my morning's routine appointments: a physical examination for a patient entering a nearby drug rehabilitation program; two different women in their thirties with high blood pressure; a young woman with a vaginal infection. About noon I finally get to Mrs. Flowers. Before entering the exam room, I read over Lenora's summary. Louise Flowers is thirty-two years old, the mother of two girls. Diagnosed four years ago as having Graves' disease, a serious hyperactivity of the thyroid gland, she was treated appropriately with continuing medication. Her husband, however, has been abusive, and Mrs. Flowers has left home several times with her two girls, Teresa and Saleena. Eventually she has always returned. Somewhere along the way, she ran out of money and stopped taking her thyroid pills. After the latest episode of abuse, she and her children went to the shelter at the Pitts Hotel, but were turned away. According to Mrs. Flowers, the staff informed her that for her to be allowed in, her husband would have to come over to the shelter and certify to the social workers that he was abusing her!

Surely Mrs. Flowers had misunderstood. Documentation (of any kind) from an abusive husband could not be a requirement for admission to a shelter for a homeless woman and her children. But when I heard similarly unbelievable tales repeated day in and day out, I began to wonder. Later that afternoon, our social worker called the shelter to get more information. She was told that the Pitts was overcrowded and that Mrs. Flowers's only option was to give her children up to Protective Services so that she could stay by herself at one of the overnight shelters for women. I don't know which story is true . . . or which represents the greater indictment of a "system" that was supposed to serve the poor. In any case, mother and daughters, aged nine and

eleven, had ended up at the large, squalid shelter for homeless adults downtown—at that time an abandoned, con-
demned building warehousing eight hundred men and
women, many of whom were actively alcoholic, drug-
addicted, or severely mentally ill.

I walk into the tiny exam room and begin the interview.
Louise is a large woman but not obese. She has, in fact, lost
weight since her thyroid started malfunctioning again. She is
anxious and is having trouble sleeping. Her pulse is rapid at
120, her skin dry, her eyes slightly bugged out. There is no
difficulty in making the diagnosis: an excess of thyroid hormone. Her lab data confirms her dangerous hyperthyroidism.
I ask Louise why she stopped taking her medicine.

"There wasn't no money," she answers, looking down at
the floor, seeming to examine her feet. "I was going to a
private doctor, but I ran up a big bill, and I couldn't pay it.
I couldn't pay for no medicine, neither." Her voice is so
soft I can barely hear it. "My husband was beating on me,
and there wasn't no money. The doctor he said he couldn't
keep seeing me if I couldn't pay. I went and got Medicaid,
but the doctor he said he didn't take that, neither. His nurse
she said go down to D.C. General or either the public
clinic. I don't know no public clinic, so I went to D.C.
General. They said I wasn't no emergency, so I'd have to
wait. I waited over six hours, and then the doctor he said
I'd have to come back to somewhere else. He didn't give
me no medicine, and I didn't want to sit there again. I can't
pay no one to take care of Saleena while I go, and I ain't
taking her down there again." She's silent for a moment. "I
knew I was getting sick."

I eventually refer her to the D.C. General Emergency
Room, where she is hospitalized for treatment. Although
Louise's condition has become—due to neglect—life-
threatening, it is medically a simple problem that could
have been avoided completely had she received medications
costing a few cents a day. Seen from the perspective of a
middle-class physician, the illness and her response to it do

not "make sense." Why can't she somehow get herself together and obtain the inexpensive medications she needs?
Why can't she stick it out at the D.C. General clinics to get
at least some level of care? But these questions ignore the
many strands of the web that binds Louise so tightly. She
suffers from a medical disease and from the real inacces-
sibility of physicians in our city; but she suffers even more
from the cumulative, battering effects of a lifetime of poverty, which have apparently rendered her incapable of using
even what minimal resources are to be had.

Gradually I began to listen differently to patients like
Mrs. Flowers. I came to realize that the distance between
my rural community in Minnesota and my new home was
virtually infinite. The stories of inner-city patients were different from the *individual* tragedies of my rural practice because they involved a kind of societal abandonment I had
not imagined possible. These were tragedies that were both
systematic and preventable. They were happening within a
nation that, I believed, had the resources to respond if only
it chose to.

The results of society's wholesale neglect became visible
every day in my office and on the streets of my neighborhood: a thirteen-year-old child, abused and in trouble herself, trying as a single mother to rear her own child; a
forty-year-old woman—whose high blood pressure had
never been adequately treated—now paralyzed from a
stroke yet unable to get disability benefits and trying to survive on $240 a month in welfare benefits; a homeless man
recently released from jail with a hernia literally the size of
a football and a knee—injured years ago and never appropriately treated—still unusable because it flailed forty-five
degrees to either side whenever he tried to put weight on it;
a three-year-old girl with vaginal gonorrhea. These lives
had been so beaten down that little was left to build upon.
Although there was certainly more to life in Washington's
ghetto neighborhoods, alcoholism, drug abuse, broken families, shattered self-images abounded.

The full impact of what I was experiencing sank in

slowly, but I soon began to feel like a medic on the front lines of a particularly bloody war, tending illnesses that were, in fact, battle wounds. But . . . what war? . . . against whom? . . . for whose sake? At first, I was both incredulous and furious that our society allowed such unnecessary suffering to exist. I had known that there was poverty in America, but I had not been prepared to find a poverty as desperate as Calcutta's in the capital of the United States!

Bernice Wardley is one of the critically wounded. She sits huddled under a blanket in a dark corner of a crowded living room at Adams House, a small shelter not far from Community of Hope. At 8:30 on an early-summer evening, it's hot and unbearably humid. Without air-conditioning in this old house, the still air pastes my shirt to my chest. The temperature in the room is at least ninety degrees, but Bernice remains buried in her blanket, not even showing her face.

The others, all men, watch me wordlessly. Except for a young white man with long, matted hair, they all look to be in their sixties, but people age quickly on the streets, and they may be fifty or less. As I cross the room toward Ms. Wardley, the men get up slowly and begin to straggle out, their eyes fastening on me as they leave. I turn toward the shape under the blanket.

"Thanks for coming over, Dr. Hilfiker," says Tina Bodner, a small, attractive woman in her early twenties who has led me into the house. She pulls the chain on the lamp by Ms. Wardley, who immediately recoils from the light. "Bernice has been here since last Tuesday, but we don't know much about her. She's been sick the whole time, but in the last few days she's gotten worse. Her temperature's 102 degrees, and she seems to be breathing pretty fast, almost heavy. She hasn't let us take her down to the emergency room, but I told her you would come over and see her here."

At the time Adams House was unique in the city, the only place where a man or woman too sick for the streets could stay for a few days or a few months. A former single-family wooden building in a run-down residential neighborhood just north of Community of Hope, the house was operated by the Community for Creative Non-Violence (CCNV). Every available space was filled with couches, beds, mats—anything that could be slept on. Fifteen, sometimes twenty, homeless, sick people were packed into various corners of the house, supervised by young volunteers.

Like many other staff members, Tina had come to join the charismatic leader of CCNV, Mitch Snyder, and live in an anarchist Christian community, finding ways to help the poor. She received only room and board in return for living with Bernice and the others and working the twelve-to-sixteen-hour days of the activist: scavenging for food, stuffing envelopes, walking on protest marches, putting in shifts at CCNV's large shelter downtown.

The house appeared chaotic. People ate and slept anywhere. Sobriety did not seem to be a requirement. There was no scheduled medical attention, just a twenty-four-hour place to stay, regular meals, and ... much caring. From time to time, one of the residents would get sicker and formal medical attention would be required. Since CCNV had no medical facilities of its own, Janelle had volunteered our group to be available for emergencies.

Kneeling next to the huddled form, Tina says gently, almost in a whisper, "Bernice, Dr. Hilfiker is here to see you."

There is no response. Her body lies completely buried within the blanket. I sit down next to her, sinking into an armchair that leaks its stuffing through several large holes in the upholstery. I bend toward her. "Hello, Ms. Wardley. I'm Dr. Hilfiker. Tina says you're sick. What seems to be the matter?"

No answer. She doesn't move or acknowledge my presence. After a few seconds I try again. "Ms. Wardley, you look like you're pretty sick. Can you tell me what's wrong?" There is a slight shake of the blanket where I imagine her head to be. She curls up more tightly. I wait perhaps two full minutes, allowing her the chance to adjust to my presence. "Are you sick, Ms. Wardley?" She changes her position and I can glimpse her head. Involuntarily, I draw back. Tina said over the phone that Ms. Wardley was forty-five years old, but she looks to be seventy, her wet gray hair plastered against a sweating black face. She steals a glance at me and averts her eyes.

"Are you sick?" I repeat, and she shakes her head again. I know she's sick, of course. The dull evening light, reinforced by the glare of the incandescent bulb, reveals the dilated stare of eyes focusing nowhere. Sweat runs down her face and she is breathing rapidly. Her mouth moves slowly, forming words without sounds. I wonder what voices she's listening to, to whom she's speaking. I sit for a few minutes searching for a path into her world.

According to Tina, Ms. Wardley lives in Georgetown, a wealthy, exclusive neighborhood in our city well known for its university basketball team and, locally, for its night life. Unlike most of the other residents of Georgetown, however, Ms. Wardley lives under a bridge in a cardboard box. She is mentally ill, most likely schizophrenic, probably paranoid. A worker at the soup kitchen where she goes for occasional meals noticed recently that she was also physically ill and tried to take her to an emergency room for medical care, but Ms. Wardley refused. She did allow herself to be cajoled into coming to Adams House, probably because she had previously known and trusted one of the volunteers.

I don't know what to do with Bernice Wardley. Her illness could be almost anything. "Ms. Wardley, I'd like to examine you to find out what's wrong. Would that be okay?" She shakes her head, tucks it more deeply into her chest, and disappears into her blanket again.

"Bernice," interrupts Tina with exaggerated gentleness, "you told me you'd let Dr. Hilfiker examine you if he came over. He can't help you unless he knows what's wrong." Tina bends down and puts her hand on her shoulder. "C'mon, Bernice. Let us help you."

There is a long, quiet moment. Then the head shakes,

and there is no further movement from underneath the blanket.

Tina stands. "I'm sorry, Dr. Hilfiker. She hasn't said three words since she got here, but I thought at least she'd let you look at her. What can we do?"

"I don't know. I can't treat her if I don't know what's going on, and I can't know that unless I can examine her. I think she needs to be in the hospital for X-rays and tests and a better examination."

"She won't go."

"I know."

Ms. Wardley certainly needs emergency hospitalization for whatever this illness is, but she also needs short-term emergency psychiatric intervention, long-term psychiatric care, a place to live, food to eat, and a loving community to nurture her. None of these is available. Like most other homeless people I care for, Ms. Wardley doesn't have Medicaid, so—even if we could convince her to accept hospitalization—neither Providence Hospital (where I have privileges) nor any of the other private hospitals in the city would accept her for anything but emergency treatment. It is most likely that her psychotic paranoia is responsible for her refusal to accept any medical treatment. This makes her, in my opinion, "a danger to herself," which should allow me as a physician to commit her for involuntary mental health treatment. But I have been through this before, with John Turnell and others. The ways in which the local laws and regulations are interpreted daily by police, psychiatric officials, and judges will allow Ms. Wardley, even in her mental state, to refuse necessary medical treatment. As to her deeper needs, she has found her way into the only place I know of that might help—a broken-down house, available only temporarily, filled to overflowing with others like her, tended by caring but overworked and untrained volunteers.

Surely, we should have been able to do *something* for this woman! I later discussed the matter with Janelle, who pointed out that I could have called the police. I could have called the Crisis Resolution Unit. Perhaps she would have been taken to the hospital and given care. But more likely she would have slipped through the net and found her way back to her cardboard box. The likely outcome of such an intervention would only have been the deepening of Ms. Wardley's paranoia and her refusal, the next time she was sick, to come even to Adams House.

In my middle-class practice in Minnesota, I would have known, probably in some detail, what happened to Ms. Wardley. She would have returned (or *been returned* by other caregivers) to my office. At the very least, I would have had feedback from others about her. But in Washington Ms. Wardley disappeared—as if in a war zone—back into the chaos of "battle." I never saw or heard of her again.

There was, I discovered over and over, a gap between what was theoretically available to the poor and what was actually accessible. There were public mental health clinics for psychotic patients; there were public health clinics for those who could not afford regular care; the emergency room at D.C. General Hospital was always there for those who could not otherwise get treated. But something almost invariably stood between theory and practice, and I kept running into it. People could cycle through the system of "care" over and over without a caring result.

It is easy to romanticize small-town life, but some of its advantages are indisputable. In my Minnesota community a family of three emotionally disabled adults who had been locked away on a farm since birth were eventually "adopted" by members of a church congregation who located housing, found sheltered jobs, and provided ongoing supervision for these "poor" people. Whenever "Crazy Jack," a patient of mine who was intermittently schizophrenic, began having his visions and acting out his paranoia, an informal committee of friends, neighbors, and helping professionals formed to respond to his mental illness, providing physical support, offering emotional encouragement, and finally arranging for temporary (even involuntary) hospitalization until he could be brought back

into the community. I could see little difference between
"Crazy Jack" and Bernice Wardley, yet in urban Washington there seemed to be no collective prepared to help our
poor who were barely treading water on their own—no one
to keep them from simply drowning.

We first discovered Leroy Solten at Pierce Shelter, a former
elementary school operated with city funds by the Council
of Churches as an overnight shelter for homeless men. At
that time Mr. Solten was thirty-nine years old, about 5′ 8″
tall, and weighed less than 110 pounds. He was obviously
ill. Mr. Solten had been discharged six weeks earlier from
D.C. General Hospital, his second hospitalization for tuberculosis (TB) within two years. Both times, after two weeks
of inpatient TB treatment, he was released "into the community" and allowed to return to the shelter system for his
"housing."

Pierce Shelter provided overnight lodging for about 150
men, many of whom were chronically ill and debilitated.
With toilets that didn't work, roaches, lice, rats, unwashed
blankets, inadequate heating, overcrowding, and a staff that
had been accused publicly of abusiveness, it was unfit for
habitation. In 1989 a District court enjoined the city from
keeping human beings in such a place. When the city did
not bring the shelter up to a minimal human standard, the
court found the city in contempt, but the shelter remained
in service without the ordered changes for an additional two
years. It was finally shut down because of budgetary constraints. As in other shelters, admission was on a first-come,
first-served basis. In other words, Mr. Solten had to wait in
line every evening for the privilege of sleeping with the
roaches. The shelter served food only once daily, a light
supper, but during the day Mr. Solten was often too weak
to walk from the shelter to a nearby store or restaurant for
other meals.

Janelle first saw Mr. Solten at the clinic on a Friday. He
was feeling worse, he said, his cough had deepened, and he
had continued to lose weight since his discharge. He'd been

drinking, so he wasn't sure how often he'd gotten his streptomycin shots, and he couldn't remember how often he was
taking his oral medications. Janelle's examination didn't
add too much to what he had told her: Mr. Solten had obviously lost a lot of weight, and his chest sounds were ab-
normal, although both findings might be chronic and not a
sign of new infection. But after finishing, Janelle was concerned that his tuberculosis might have become active
again.

Tuberculosis is a serious, difficult-to-treat communicable
infection of the lungs and (sometimes) other parts of the
body. It usually spreads from one person to another through
droplets that are coughed, sneezed, or breathed out of the
lungs. It is the classic "tragic" disease (the famous "consumption" of nineteenth-century opera), once much feared.
During the last several decades, however, with powerful
new antibiotics available, tuberculosis could have been for
all practical purposes eradicated in the United States, had
all cases been properly treated. Unfortunately, because of
the length of time required to destroy all tuberculosis germs
in an infected patient, the bacillus that causes the infection
can undergo mutations and become drug-resistant if the patient does not take his or her medications according to a
precise schedule. It is in homeless men like Mr. Solten—
who frequently cannot or do not take their medications as
directed—that new strains of tuberculosis resistant to any
known drugs are most likely to be incubated. Those strains
of TB can then be passed on to others.

This is not merely a theoretical risk. It is now not unusual to find tuberculosis strains resistant to three, four, or
even five of the most commonly used medications. Tuberculosis among those with AIDS—a common mix of diseases, especially in the shelters—is even more difficult to
treat because the patient's immune system cannot assist the
medications. In such cases, the emergence of resistant
strains becomes even more probable. Health professionals
no longer consider the eradication of tuberculosis from this
country a realistic possibility; on the contrary, they foresee

a developing epidemic. The potential implications—even for healthy, affluent people, to say nothing of those whose health is marginal—are staggering. A first step to avert the epidemic would be to make sure that patients follow the prescribed regimen.

In the District of Columbia, tuberculosis patients who cannot arrange for private care are followed at the city's Area C Chest Clinic after they are discharged from the hospital. During the first months of treatment, more seriously ill patients often require intramuscular injections of streptomycin several times a week and so must come repeatedly to this single clinic from all over the city. Thereafter—for a period lasting from nine to eighteen months—the patient returns monthly, and the clinic dispenses enough of each of the needed oral anti-tuberculosis medications to last until the next visit. It is, however, the task of the clinic to monitor the patients and of its outreach team to stay in touch with and treat those who cannot or will not comply with treatment plans. That, at least, is the theory.

Janelle called Area C to ascertain Mr. Solten's status: How sick had he been in the hospital? What medications was he supposed to be taking? Had the outreach nurse found him for each of his needed streptomycin injections? But no one answering the phone at Area C that Friday afternoon even knew if a Mr. Solten was being followed by the clinic, much less had answers for Janelle's questions. If anyone was going to provide him with help before the start of the business day on Monday, Janelle would have to arrange it. The first priority became making sure he had food over the weekend. Sister Lenora, at that time working as an outreach nurse for SOME (So Others May Eat), the third clinic in our loosely affiliated group, caught him at the Pierce Shelter early Saturday, Sunday, and Monday mornings by arriving just before 7:00 A.M., when all the men had to leave for the day. She checked on his physical status, made sure he was taking the medications that he had with him, and provided him with some food. On Monday, Janelle again called Area C. It turned out that Area C *did* have an active file on Mr. Solten that, for some reason, had not been accessible the previous Friday afternoon. An outreach worker, Janelle was told, should be going out three times a week to give him his shots.

Janelle reported her concern that Mr. Solten looked quite sick and needed medical attention. If the outreach worker was making contact with him three times a week, Janelle did not understand how a trained medical professional could have missed seeing that he needed immediate attention. She requested that the outreach worker visit him that day, not only to give him his shot but also to determine whether he needed more intensive medical evaluation. The worker who came, however, did not take him back to Area C for further medical evaluation but simply gave him his streptomycin injection, despite the fact that Mr. Solten—if his tuberculosis had again become active—posed an immediate risk to the other men at the shelter. Finally, after Janelle called a second time to complain, Mr. Solten was taken back to Area C for evaluation, only to be discharged that same day to Adams House, which was full—as always—of homeless people even more ill than those at Pierce Shelter.

A week later, Mr. Solten developed a fever of 104 degrees and was hospitalized at D.C. General Hospital. Active, contagious tuberculosis was diagnosed—for the third time.

Mr. Solten's was hardly a singular case. It is routine for homeless TB patients who have been admitted to either private or public hospitals to be treated as inpatients for a week or two and then discharged to the shelters, to be supervised by Area C Chest Clinic. From a purely medical viewpoint, this plan seems perfectly reasonable. After a patient receives two weeks of adequate, multidrug treatment, the droplets he or she coughs, sneezes, or breathes into the air no longer contain the tuberculosis bacilli, so the patient is no longer contagious, no longer a danger to anyone else. Outpatient treatment then becomes appropriate.

Unfortunately, the medically reasonable becomes inappropriate in light of the particular needs of the homeless population, whose lack of predictable daily routine makes a regular, long-term medical regimen almost impossible to follow. As might be expected, many homeless individuals like Mr. Solten are severely malnourished and under great physical stress; many others are alcoholic, mentally ill, or sick with AIDS. The inevitable result is that either the patient does not comply with recommended treatment or— even if he or she does—the drug regimen that works on otherwise healthy, well-nourished adults proves ineffective. And the interventions of clinics like Area C prove in practice to be merely stopgaps, at best inadequate and at worst irresponsible. All too often, within months the still-infected patients are again coughing up the contagious bacilli.

To complicate matters further, homeless men like Mr. Solten are typically discharged to a crowded shelter— almost by definition in Washington, if you say "shelter," you mean "crowded"—where they sleep, dormitory-style, in rooms of eight to ten chronically ill and debilitated persons. These are perfect conditions for the spread of TB and other infectious diseases. Researchers in Boston have found that almost half of the people who have been in large city shelters for over two years have a positive skin test indicating infection with tuberculosis.[3] Over a one- or two-year period, Janelle saw as patients at least ten men in the shelters who had to be readmitted to the hospital for further treatment of their *recurrent* tuberculosis and were then discharged for a third or fourth time to the shelters, where the process began all over again.

Now that Mr. Solten had been admitted for the third time to D.C. General Hospital, Janelle was quite reasonably apprehensive that after initial treatment he would be released into yet another shelter. She talked with the chief of the medical service to which Mr. Solten was assigned, who confirmed that the patient would indeed have to be discharged once he was no longer "contagious." Hospital beds were sorely needed for the acutely ill. Possible or even probable noncompliance with treatment could not justify, said the hospital doctor, inpatient care for the nine to eighteen months of required treatment. It was neither the hospital's role nor a responsible use of scarce resources to provide long-term care. The doctor was sympathetic and concerned, but there was, she said, really nothing she could do.

Janelle's only remaining option was to convince an appropriate public health officer to take legal measures to require Mr. Solten to stay at Montebello Pulmonary Rehabilitation Unit, a long-term sanitarium in Baltimore for which the District of Columbia would have to pay the daily rate. The health official with that authority, however, refused to consider such commitment, reassuring Janelle that D.C. General would be notified to keep Mr. Solten until an appropriate disposition was worked out. Two weeks later, of course, that "disposition" turned out to be Mr. Solten's discharge to a public shelter.

One "Mr. Solten" followed another into my office at Community of Hope, and for so few of them could I alone or Community of Hope alone offer any but the most palliative help—often allowing people to recuperate barely long enough to reenter the full misery of their lives "out there." I had tried to prepare myself for this, but there had been limits to the horrors I could imagine, which bore little relation to the seemingly limitless realities of the street.

When I first entered this universe of visible suffering, I assumed that provoking political change was just a matter of getting the ordinary, everyday people around me to understand what was happening; then—as had been true for "Crazy Jack" and others in Minnesota—there would be an outpouring of money and concern for the welfare of the poor. But as I saw homeless men with feet black, oozing, and gangrenous from frostbite discharged from emergency rooms; as hospital social workers threatened to discharge elderly demented men back to the streets; as alcoholics seeking help at the city detoxification center were turned away "because they weren't drunk enough"; as child protection workers dragged their feet or refused outright to investigate abusive situations we reported—I began to realize that the poverty I was seeing was much deeper than I could have imagined. Apparently the homelessness, the lack of medical attention, the malnutrition, the staggering infant mortality rate had been in some way *accepted.* They had become "tolerable evils." It would not be enough to inform people of what was happening. In some sense they already knew, and were numbed to it.

It is not surprising, of course, that "community" is so much more difficult to fashion within a large city. In contemporary rural areas or small towns—whether the community chooses to respond to the neediness or not—the very needy generally remain in manageable ratio to the *capacity* of the community to care. The urban ghettoizing of the poor, however, brings such large numbers of the needy to a small geographic location that the ratio tips and the community's capacity to care is overwhelmed. At this point the all-too-understandable response is for compassion to shut down.

Chapter 4

TRAILBLAZING

The chaos of the inner city would have been impossibly frustrating had I not been part of a community committed both to social justice and to a spirituality that emphasized reconciliation between rich and poor. Marja and I had come to Washington to be a part of the Church of the Saviour, founded in 1947 at the initiative of Reverend Gordon Cosby. As a military chaplain, Gordon had been struck by how little impact church membership seemed to have had on the day-to-day lives of his military "parishioners." Upon his return from duty, he and several others began building a church community in which the "outward journey" of mission would have an importance equal to the "inward journey" of prayer and devotion. Today the church's doctrine is ecumenical: The finer points of theology and history that tend to separate church bodies one from another are not considered as important as the creation of structures that make the essentials of a Christian life possible. Although there are currently nine different worshiping communities of ten to twenty-five members each within the church, its fundamental unit is the "mission group"—two to ten people coming together to develop and support a particular project. Each church member must participate in a mission group, meeting weekly for study, personal sharing, and the project's work. At any given time there will be approximately fifty mission groups operating within the church, averaging three or four members each. Members also commit themselves to an hour daily of prayer, silence, and study; to weekly worship with the community; to "proportional giving" to the missions of the church and to the poor (ten percent of gross income is the minimum, but the percentage rises as income rises); and to two silent weekend retreats a year.

Christ House began the way so many Church of the Saviour missions did: Someone saw a need and called on others to help her respond to it. One afternoon Robert Jones, a middle-aged homeless man, came off the streets and into the clinic at SOME. It was winter, rainy and cold. He had rain-soaked shoes but no socks, a lightweight jacket with no shirt underneath, no gloves or hat. He was cold, wet, and hungry. He had been coughing for some weeks and was now feeling worse: feverish and weak. Janelle believed he had bronchitis but was concerned he might also have pneumonia or even tuberculosis. She and the clinic staff fed him, clothed him, warmed him, and then spent much of the afternoon trying to get him a chest X-ray or, even better, admission to a hospital. But of course Robert had neither insurance nor Medicaid, and he was probably not sick enough to qualify for emergency hospital admission (which must, by law, be provided regardless of finances). Obtaining the needed lab work and X-rays for indigent patients, however, is a complicated and time-consuming business, and—despite Janelle's attempts—it could not be completed before the lab's five o'clock closing.

Eventually Robert was given some antibiotics and instructions to return in the morning so that further arrangements could be made. It was now early evening. Robert was weak and probably slow. He didn't make it back to the shelter he'd been staying at until too late. His bed had been given away, and he was left to fend for himself on the streets. The next morning Robert was found frozen to death in a telephone booth.

Robert—and others like him—convinced Janelle of the need for a place for homeless people too sick to be on the streets but not sick enough to qualify for emergency hospital care. Not only were there individuals like Robert who needed temporary help while other arrangements were being made, but homeless patients were too often being discharged from hospitals as if they had a home to go to, while others could not be admitted in the first place because their diseases either did not really warrant hospital care or, like Robert's, were "not severe enough" to demand the emergency admission available for the indigent. It is difficult to recuperate from even a relatively minor illness in a shelter that provides no meals and closes for the day at seven in the morning. Leg ulcers, frostbitten feet, broken limbs, pneumonia, and countless other diseases require a level of rest and care hardly possible in a shelter—or on the streets. How, for instance, does one manage diarrhea after the shelter closes and one must spend the day where there are no public toilets? People like Robert needed a permanent home; or, if that was not available, at least a place to live while they were recuperating. Adams House—small, unequipped, understaffed, and for all practical purposes unfunded—was hardly enough.

In the fall of 1983, a wealthy friend of the church who had been impressed by its commitment to justice for the poor made available a $2.5 million gift to create an infirmary for the homeless. At the same time, a vacant, decaying apartment building across the street from Columbia Road Health Services went up for sale. We had noticed it before. Homeless people often crawled through its half-boarded-up windows and slept there. On its front steps was a more-or-less permanent encampment of homeless Cuban refugees, first deposited in the United States in the early 1980s by the Mariel Boat Lift by means of which Castro had shipped several thousand prisoners and psychiatric patients to the shores of Florida. Columbia Road, the central thoroughfare of the Adams-Morgan neighborhood, less than a mile from Belmont Street, had been undergoing an urban renewal of sorts, and this building was the only one still boarded up. We purchased it early in 1984.

Janelle and Allen "called" the Christ House Mission Group, and five of us—Marja and I, Don and Ellen Martin, and Sister Marcella Jordan, a social worker at Columbia Road Health Services—responded. Beginning in the spring of 1984, the seven of us met every Sunday evening according to the usual mission group practice. We shared a meal, worshiped, studied together, and planned for Christ House. The early meetings were exhilarating. The dream was to build not only an infirmary for homeless men but also a community in which rich and poor could live together. We knew of no similar community in which doctors lived with their patients, but for inspiration we studied Dorothy Day's Catholic Worker communities (houses of hospitality for the homeless, operated by groups of people who live in those houses) as well as Jean Vanier's L'Arche communities (small houses for mentally handicapped individuals living with mentally normal assistants). Very quickly two important questions arose: How closely would we, the staff, live with each other? How intimately would we live with the homeless patients whom we were inviting?

Like, I suspect, the Goetcheuses, the Martins, and Sister Marcella, Marja and I secretly harbored the dream of living in community with the homeless persons who would be our patients. Our worst nightmare, I suppose, was that the same dream would come true! I wasn't even sure I wanted to live in such close proximity with the others in the mission group, much less with strangers from the street. I'm an introvert. I need my own private spaces. I have a powerful desire for order—my own kind of order. My early experiences with the seemingly bottomless needs of my patients at Community of Hope made me fearful of opening myself so completely to my patients. Besides, what were we to do about drunkenness, violence, drug addiction, if it came into our own homes? We quickly realized that living together as one household was not a feasible alternative, even for the mission group.

At the same time, all of us wanted to leave open the possibility of growing into such a community in the future.

With the help of a professional architect, we began to draw up plans. The first two floors of Christ House would be set aside for our patients: bedrooms—both individual and dormitory-style, to accommodate up to thirty-four residents—nursing station, exam rooms, kitchen, dining room, activity rooms, and offices. The third and fourth floors would include separate apartments for those of us who planned to live and work there, a larger community room, a small chapel, and six small, motel-style rooms for guests (mostly volunteers who would come for varying lengths of time).

Initially it seemed hard to justify using half of a building purchased for the express purpose of serving the poor as living space for ourselves, who could afford to live elsewhere. But each of us sensed that Christ House would be more than just another institution for the poor. Without quite being able to articulate why, we believed that whatever degree of community was created by our living situation would be at least as important as the medical healing that took place. We hoped that our initial plans for Christ House would prove a way station to a closer "living with" the poor.

We were not, of course, going to live *with* the poor, exactly. Our living space would be the entire third and fourth floors, which were to be "off limits" for the men living below. Keys and coded locks would keep them out. They would have dormitory-style bedrooms for two to eight men, while we had comfortable, multibedroom apartments with as much privacy as we wanted. They would eat in a common dining hall; we would each have our own kitchens. In addition to the common front entrance off Columbia Road, a separate "residential entrance" along the side of the building (protected, again, by locks and coded gates) would allow us and our personal guests private access to our apartments. We believed that our decision to live in the same building with the men was an important one, but it did not resolve the continuing tension between our current address in the middle class and our assumed destination—

which, in some way we still could not define, would include the homeless men living downstairs. Demolition of the decaying interior of the old building began in the last part of 1984. None of us had ever been involved in a project of such magnitude. Watching the building take shape week by week was exciting, but—because of perpetual construction delays—frustrating. First our contractor promised us an early autumn finish. Then we were assured "absolutely" that we would be able to move in by November 1, and we gave notice to our respective landlords for December 1. By mid-November it was obvious the building would not be ready in time, so we settled for having the third and fourth floors finished first. Over the long Thanksgiving weekend of 1985, the seven of us in the mission group (along with the three Goetcheus children and the three Hilfiker children) moved in. On Sunday, December 1, in place of our regular mission group worship, we proceeded by candlelight through each of the rooms of the still darkened and unfinished Christ House, asking God's blessing on the work to come.

Construction wasn't finished when Mr. Malloy was discharged from the hospital in mid-December, but because we had promised to open our doors by Christmas and even scheduled a Christmas Eve worship service, we accepted him anyway. Three doctors and their families lived upstairs; anticipating that we would begin with eight to ten patients, we had already hired a staff of nurses and their aides. Volunteers from the church were anxious to help. Kitchen construction wasn't completed, so those of us in residence took turns cooking food for our first guest, bringing meals to him three times a day on trays.

Mr. Malloy was in his late sixties, a small black man with closely cropped white hair. He'd been hospitalized with an irregular heartbeat, and he needed to recuperate. Although he never really questioned us, Mr. Malloy was clearly overwhelmed by all the attention he was receiving; that he got the rest he needed is doubtful. Although the hospital social worker had told us Mr. Malloy was "homeless," we soon discovered that, while the term was literally accurate, his actual situation was a more complicated one. His wife had recently died, and soon after he'd required hospital admission. While there, he couldn't keep up the rent and lost his apartment. The social worker could find no adequate placement for him, so—acting on behalf of her patient in order to find him a decent situation—she didn't give us quite the full story. At our official opening, while we worshiped in the yet-incomplete dining room downstairs and held to our exalted dreams of a medical recovery shelter for street people, a solitary, elderly gentleman who had never lived on the street in the first place and was probably too harassed to do much recovering among us, sat in his bed upstairs. Mr. Malloy, with his kindhearted and good-humored acceptance of our perhaps comical ministrations did, however, provide us with a gentle entry into our work.

When construction was finally completed, our patients began coming to us directly from the streets, from the shelters, from hospital emergency rooms, and on discharge from hospitals. It was early January 1986, and among our first patients were men with frostbitten fingers and toes, as well as others with third-degree burns on their backs from having slept without adequate protection on steam grates downtown. Men came for the treatment of tuberculosis and other respiratory diseases, cancer, heart disease, strokes, fractures, gunshot and stab wounds. Others came to recuperate for a few days from colds, flus, sore throats, skin infestations, or diarrhea. Still others came because there was simply no other place to go: schizophrenic older men who needed to be off the streets; burned-out alcoholics not really interested in stopping drinking but feeling too poorly to continue. We had hoped to move slowly, to give us all a chance to adjust to our new situation, but by the end of January we were already caring for eighteen patients at a time and beginning to feel the stress.

We had not originally envisioned homeless women as patients at Christ House and had not, therefore, drawn separate facilities into our architectural plans. This exclusion was originally more by default than a conscious decision. At the time virtually all care for the homeless was segregated by sex; even the few shelters that admitted both women and men kept them separated on different floors or in different wings. We hardly considered anything else. As plans became reality, however, Sister Loreta Jordan, a recent addition to the mission group, began to challenge our original decision and lobbied for us to admit women. Perhaps because we had up to that point made all decisions by consensus and did not want to look too closely at potentially irreconcilable differences, we had never fully debated the pros and cons of the issue. (In fact, on joining the group, Loreta had not even been aware of the men-only decision.) In 1986, it was clear that the need for a medical recovery shelter was less desperate for women than for men: The population of homeless women was considerably smaller, and most of the women's shelters stayed open during the day and offered a higher level of care. Unlike the men, women who became sick had a place where they could stay in bed and recuperate.

What was less clear—but what the majority of us in the mission group nevertheless firmly believed—was that homeless women were, on the average, simply more difficult to care for than men. This was common wisdom among shelter providers at the time. Women tended to have run through more support systems before they became homeless than did the men. Families and friends would still, as a rule, bend over backward—in ways they often would not for men—to keep a woman from becoming homeless. The fear, then, was that the women who ended up on the streets were the ones least able to get along with others. And, in fact, a much greater percentage of homeless women than men were severely mentally ill.

We decided, for all these reasons, to restrict the population of Christ House to males. But we continued to feel uncomfortable with our decision, and the muted disagreement within the mission group persisted. Shortly after we opened, Janelle decided to try admitting a few women, one at a time, to see how it would go. The first two women were carefully selected, and things went well. Then came Lizzy.

Elizabeth McIntyre was an elderly psychotic white woman whose untamed white hair matched her spirit. Her physical illness was not severe, but her deep bronchial coughing made her sound as if she were dying. The director of the shelter at which Lizzy was staying feared they wouldn't be able to handle her. So Lizzy moved into Christ House . . . and quickly took over. Lizzy knew what she wanted (even if, in her disordered mind, what she wanted changed from minute to minute), and she would yell loudly from her room every few minutes or parade half-dressed, her bathrobe usually open and flowing behind her, through the hall to the nursing station until she got it—despite the bed rest prescribed for her recuperation. Lizzy was also a smoker. She was unable to go outside, refused to join the men in the TV room where smoking was allowed, and insisted on lighting up in bed despite the house prohibition. The nurses began to complain that they couldn't cope with her. When she set her hair on fire, we decided we'd had enough. Obviously one unpleasantly psychotic woman would not precipitate a men-only policy, but Lizzy confirmed our prejudices, and we were only too happy to revert to our original intent: Christ House would be a medical recovery shelter for homeless men—which left us with problems enough.

Some of those problems were, of course, medical. Though many of the staff already had experience in health care for the indigent, one never quite gets used to the mix of challenges that emerge in medical care for the homeless. There is comparatively little geriatric care (a surprising percentage of a normal primary-care practice) because so few homeless people live to old age. Their life expectancy seems to be about twenty years less than that of the average middle-class person. Permanent physical deformities are common, often the result of poor or absent medical care: a broken leg not properly set, a congenitally dislocated hip never treated, a leg amputated because of diabetes in a fifty-year-old man who had no place to store his insulin and whose needles kept being stolen at the shelter. Wounds from serious injuries are common at Christ House: gunshot wounds; broken bones from attacks suffered while sleeping in abandoned buildings; multiple injuries from run-ins with cars. Even routine medical problems—diabetes, heart disease, stroke—are vastly complicated by poverty and homelessness.

But these medical problems, while frequently severe, were not the primary cause of the distress that we as a staff soon began to feel. We knew what to do for the medical diseases, which we took care of as we had been doing in our clinics for several years. But in those clinics, when the appointment was over, the patient disappeared until his or her next visit. Certainly, providing medical care in the office to an alcoholic who is trying to detox can be difficult, for example. Once he or she leaves the clinic, however, one moves on to the next patient; at night, one goes home. At Christ House it was different.

"David, Mr. Melendez just attacked Walter Williams with his crutch."

I'm at the office at Community of Hope, and it's Ann Richards, the director of nursing at Christ House on the phone. I take a deep breath. "What happened?" I ask. "Has he been drinking?"

George Melendez, one of the Cuban refugees who used to hang out on the steps of the abandoned building that became Christ House, was my patient. I'd admitted him a week earlier on discharge from the hospital: He'd broken his leg and was going to need five more weeks in a walking cast. I knew that Mr. Melendez was an alcoholic, but he'd been working to stay dry. I also suspected he might have some psychiatric illness, perhaps a personality disorder; but I didn't really know. His English was limited and I spoke no Spanish. Assessing the subtleties of psychiatric symptoms through a translator is a questionable process at best, and diagnosis was often a gross approximation. A deportee with the Mariel Boat Lift, Mr. Melendez naturally had no record of his medical history.

"I don't think he's been drinking. Walter has, though. He came in drunk this morning and, according to Marie, started picking on George. I guess Walter didn't actually take the first swing, but Marie said he was responsible for starting it. Don told me to discharge Walter, and I have. What do you want me to do with Mr. Melendez?"

We were just starting up, and our rules hadn't been worked out yet. We knew we could tolerate neither alcohol nor violence, so either had been made grounds for expulsion. I was only slightly acquainted with Walter Williams, but I'd seen him rile others up, even when he wasn't drunk. Although Mr. Melendez had been working hard to cooperate with us, I knew he had a short fuse. I could well imagine Walter igniting it. If Marie, one of the aides, had seen the fight and thought it Walter's fault, was it fair to throw Mr. Melendez out? With Walter gone, George was little risk to anyone else; but wasn't sticking to our rules important, too?

"We'd probably better kick him out, Ann."

"I suppose so, but with his leg like that, I don't know where he can go."

"Well, maybe we should think about it then," I said, hesitating. "Did Loreta have a chance to talk with him?" Sister Loreta was his social worker, and I hoped she might know a place to which we could transfer him. "Is she around?"

"I think she talked with him, but she didn't say anything to me. She's out now, anyway."

"Oh well, ask her to call me when she gets in, or I'll find her myself."

As often happened, I got swept up in my work at Community of Hope and forgot to call Loreta. It was evening, after I'd returned to Christ House and stopped at the nurses' station on the way to our apartment, before I remembered Mr. Melendez. I called Loreta in her fourth-floor apartment.

"What do you think we should do with Mr. Melendez?" I asked.

"I don't know, David." She sighed. "Our rules say any violence and you're out, but this doesn't really seem like his fault. Walter was really drunk and obnoxious. I didn't actually see it, but Marie said that Walter goaded George. George has a temper, of course, but I don't think he'll hurt anyone else. Besides, he looked so repentant when I talked with him, like a little puppy dog. He's afraid of being kicked out."

"I don't want to throw him out, either," I said, "but we have to let the men know they're safe in here. We haven't had any other violence, and I think that's because people know they'll get kicked out if they start anything . . . or even if they don't start it. I don't know what to do with George, but I'm more worried about the effect of the precedent on the other men."

"Yes, I know what you mean. On the other hand, all the men know who really started it, and he *did* get kicked out."

"Well, maybe. Let me talk with Janelle. I'll get back to you."

I called Janelle, who was inclined, as always, to give the patient the benefit of the doubt. But in this case she wasn't sure. I called Don in his apartment and talked with him, too. He also saw both sides of the picture. I eventually decided that we would let Mr. Melendez off with a stern warning.

I had just spent over two hours of what was supposed to be my time off dealing with Mr. Melendez. The issue was hardly "medical," but it was typical of the kind of thing that sapped our time and energy, frayed our nerves, and divided our group. Mr. Melendez stayed, but some staff members were still upset that we had flouted our agreed-upon rules. Eventually, after considerable discussion, which required even more time, we decided again that *any* violence, provoked or not, would be grounds for discharge. The rule was a good one, I think, and in part responsible for our experiencing so little violence during the following years.

Other rules were established through the same messy

process of provisional decision, modification by experience, and final codification—though that, too, could be modified. We decided on a 9 P.M. curfew without much difficulty, since almost all the city shelters had a similar rule, but we rarely discharged a patient simply for violating the curfew. Since patient circumstances varied so greatly, we were never able to define a limit to the permissible length of stay, though one month became about average. The principle of no alcohol or drug use was easy to agree upon, but it was far harder to find consensus about how to enforce it. What was to be the basis for determining drug or alcohol use: behavioral changes? alcohol on the breath? a blood or urine test? Who was to be responsible for blowing the whistle: aides, who frequently had close relationships with the patients? or the evening nurse, who might start feeling like a suspicious ogre? Were there to be any exceptions? Were we to discharge a patient who returned to Christ House with a "slight" smell of alcohol on his breath two days prior to his appointment, which we'd spent weeks arranging, with a medical specialist? I argued for strict enforcement—but sometimes I found myself bending the rules for one of my own patients.

Caught in an infraction of the rules, the men sometimes complained that the lack of consistent enforcement led to confusion about the nature of the rules themselves . . . and they had a point. We lumbered forward as best we could.

We took pride in the well-kept look and friendly atmosphere of Christ House. Jimilu Mason, a member of the church and an established sculptor, created a bronze figure of the kneeling Jesus, slightly larger than life, which quickly became the focal point of the tiny plaza in front of the building: Neighborhood children could hardly pass by without climbing all over it. A cluster of patients seemed always to be sitting in front of the building, chatting and laughing, often calling out to passersby. First-time visitors often commented on how clean and modern the interior of the building seemed and on the artwork that decorated the walls—by both professional artists and former patients. On the ground floor was a shower room where men arriving from the shelters—inevitably filthy and infested with lice—could clean themselves up before receiving a fresh set of clothes from the nearby "clothes closet." Just off the main hallway of the ground floor were a large, comfortable living room, a completely equipped institutional kitchen, and a pleasant dining room that served as a meeting area. The second floor—which perhaps looked a bit too much like a hospital—had two eight-bed wards at the end of the hall, a nurses' station, probably overly sterile patient rooms with hospital beds, and a television room. But even on this floor patients were typically up and about, in wheelchairs or on crutches. The TV room was filled with patients, who often engaged in loud running commentary on whatever was on the screen, and the glass-enclosed "sun room" (constructed from the shell of the former building's front porch) gave the place an almost festive mood. In addition to the regular staff, volunteers mingled with the patients and performed a variety of tasks, from serving meals to teaching art or poetry classes, from sorting clothes to entering computer data for our full-time fund-raiser. A certain amount of cheerful confusion was the norm.

Amid all this, the staff managed to establish a pleasant and well-ordered routine in our daily existence. In fact, our life upstairs was remarkably little affected by the chaotic lives of the men, only one floor below. Occasionally, lying awake at night, I could hear loud voices arguing in the eight-bed room directly beneath us, but whenever the men stopped me on my way upstairs to ask a question, medical or otherwise, they were quite deferential. Since the medical work downstairs mostly involved nursing care rather than the technical diagnosis and treatment for which a doctor might be required, I was rarely called at night; besides, I shared calls with Don and Janelle, which lightened the burden even more. I came to feel less threatened by the men downstairs than I had been by the telephone in Minnesota. Sometimes the lives on the floor below did interfere with

our life . . . although not always in the ways I had worried
about. Alcohol was strictly forbidden for patients at Christ
House, but no such rule applied to us on the third and
fourth floors. The liquor store across the street was in plain
view of the large windows of the men's sun room, so Marja
or I usually walked a discreet distance to a liquor store farther down Columbia Road to do our shopping. We were
careful to bring our purchases home through the side door,
a residential entrance where we would not be confronted by
a patient. I once walked home with two six-packs of beer
in the bottom of a plain brown bag that looked, as far as I
could tell, like any other sack of groceries. For once I decided to use the front entrance and walk up the stairs; but
I felt not unlike a teenager returning home, furtively chew-
ing on mints to hide the smell of alcohol. A man I hardly
knew was going out as I came in. "Whatcha got in the bag,
Doc?" he asked. Bruce Lee, one of my patients and a recovering alcoholic, found me in the stairway: "That bag
looks a little heavy, Doc. Need some help carrying it?"
Both men had that slight smile on their lips and look in
their eyes that said: "I know what's in that bag." (*How* they
knew I have no idea.) From then on, I went through the
back parking lot and the residential entrance when I
brought my beer home.

It quickly became clear that when Christ House "worked,"
it could work miracles. Lincoln Pearson was one of our
early patients. He had been in construction work until he
lost his job following industry-wide layoffs in 1981. For the
next several years he tried to live on his savings while caring for a brother with lung cancer. When the brother died
in 1983, Mr. Pearson moved in with his niece, but "we got
to disagreeing about things," and in the fall of 1985 he
found himself on the street, sleeping at what was probably
the best shelter in the city, Union Gospel Mission.

    Even before becoming homeless, Mr. Pearson could not
afford medical care for his diabetes, so "I wouldn't go to
the clinic until something drastic happened." For a while he

continued his insulin shots, but it's almost impossible to store medications and supplies properly when living on the streets. One of the feared complications of diabetes is ulceration of the feet. The sores can begin as routine blisters, cuts, or even ingrown toenails. Since diabetes can gradually destroy the nerves to the legs, a growing numbness may keep the patient from noticing the sores because they don't hurt—especially if they are out of sight on the underside of the foot. Diabetes also causes poor circulation, which makes healing very slow, even if the sores are noticed and cared for properly. The tiniest cut or the simplest blister, left untreated, can turn into an infected and dangerous ulceration. Because Mr. Pearson had to walk or stand so much of the day, his feet became swollen, compromising his circulation even further.

Quite frequently the sores on the surface of the skin don't look very bad to an untrained observer, but Mr. Pearson's finally became so noticeable that even *he* felt something "drastic" was happening to him and went to the emergency room at D.C. General. When the dead skin on one foot was cut away, large areas of gangrene were exposed just beneath the skin. He was hospitalized immediately. After an unsuccessful monthlong battle to save the foot, however, his physicians finally recommended amputation of the left leg just below the knee.

Beyond his initial recovery, Mr. Pearson needed time for the amputation to heal, the stump to be shaped, and a prosthesis to be molded. He also needed weekly trips to D.C. General for surgical follow-up, physical therapy, and the fitting of the prosthesis—all difficult for a one-legged man recently discharged from the hospital to manage from a shelter. A nursing home bed for an indigent patient would not be available for months. Christ House had just opened, and Mr. Pearson became one of our early guests.

For people like Mr. Pearson who require only time for healing and convalescing, much of the rehabilitation at Christ House is provided by volunteer effort. Mr. Pearson found an art class taught by a volunteer and began painting for the first time in his life. Some weeks later his paintings hung on the first-floor walls. Because his medical problem required months of surgical follow-up and physical therapy, Mr. Pearson stayed at Christ House considerably longer than the one-month average. He involved himself actively in a Bible study group of which he eventually became the leader, and he was later discharged to one of three Samaritan Inns—another Church of the Saviour project, comprising small, transitional group homes where (over the course of several months to a year) homeless men can stabilize themselves, find employment, and, it is hoped, move back into society. After fourteen months, Mr. Pearson was accepted at Sarah's Circle—yet another of the church's projects—which provides permanent housing for the elderly poor. Five years after the amputation of his leg, Mr. Pearson sits on the Board of Directors of both Sarah's Circle and Columbia Road Health Services, continues to paint (he and his artwork have been featured in the *Washington Post*), and plays an active part in the life of our community.

Mr. Pearson, of course, is a "success story." Although over half of the men who enter Christ House are eventually discharged back to a hospital, a treatment program, a halfway house, a community residence facility, a nursing home, or even in some few cases to an apartment of their own, many simply go back to the streets; and many of those discharged to a placement of some sort return fairly quickly to the streets, anyway. One of the contradictions of life at Christ House is our discharging back to the streets men who have, we say, "become like family" when their temporary illness is no longer acute enough to require our care—even though most have long-term problems (alcoholism, drug addiction, diabetes, heart conditions, cancer, AIDS) and would obviously be much better off either moving into a permanent and caring home or staying with us. Christ House is a halfway measure, imperfect, just a beginning . . . and that remains true even now that it has grown into a relatively large organization.°

Other contradictions complicated our effort to live as a community. On the one hand, despite the locked doors, the coded elevator to the third floor, and the separate residential entrance, we did in a certain sense live with—at least, in daily contact with—the homeless men downstairs. Most of the time we came in through the first-floor hallways, often stopping to chat at the second-floor nurses' station. Marja taught some of the men at Academy of Hope (the small adult-education school for basic literacy and high-school-equivalency exam [GED] preparation that she founded and directed) or tutored them downstairs. She and the girls would sometimes volunteer to serve food in the kitchen, getting to know the men that way. My son, Kai—six when we moved in—treated the rest of Christ House as his little village. We didn't have a television set in our apartment, but he quickly discovered those downstairs and took up the position of house mascot, playing cards, chess, or Ping-Pong with anyone who was willing. We would go to the semiannual talent show, where the girls and I would sing and play the guitar. When regular Sunday-morning worship services began downstairs in the dining room, we would sometimes attend, sitting next to men who were my pa-

---

° With a yearly budget of over a million dollars, Christ House now employs full-time registered nurses to work in the second-floor infirmary around the clock, a permanent administrative staff that occupies the few small offices on the first floor, and full-time cooks who (along with dozens of volunteers) provide three meals a day from a large, well-equipped kitchen. Christ House receives a little less than half its yearly budget as a grant from the city's Commission on Social Services. The remainder arrives mostly in the form of gifts from individuals, although charitable foundations contribute significantly. Volunteers, church groups, and other organizations donate time, clothes, and food. The social workers, nurses, doctors, and counselors contribute to the financial viability of Christ House by taking salaries significantly lower than they might find elsewhere. There is never a surplus of funds, but somehow there always seems to be enough to meet payroll and begin to dream of new work.

tients. No longer faceless figures on the street, the men became for us real people with real identities.

But these contacts hardly made us one with the men downstairs. We are not poor, and—barring misfortune outside our control—we will never experience their sort of poverty, not even if we were to choose it deliberately. We are irredeemably middle class. We live within blocks of the poorest neighborhood in the city, but—when our benefits are added in—Marja's and my combined income approaches $50,000 a year. My children live in a shelter for homeless men, but they have their own rooms and attend the best schools in the city. During the day I work in the midst of people who have virtually nothing, but at night I return to the safety and comfort of our apartment, separated from the men downstairs by locks and codes—not to mention a set of middle-class experiences and expectations so deeply and mysteriously locked and encoded in me as to make me profoundly alien to the poor I work with . . . and vice versa. Yes, I work with the poor, but I have not begun to join them.

What is more, I never will. There are privileges of birth and upbringing I could never renounce, even if I wanted to. I could give away all of my money, but none of my education. No matter how poor I became, I would always have the possibility of returning to the mainstream and beginning again. I could renounce the trappings of privilege and live in a tenement, forfeit my health insurance and give away my retirement income, but—were I ever in desperate need—my parents or my mother-in-law or my siblings or my church community or my friends (all with solid, middle-class resources) would be present to bail me out. No matter how poor I became, I would always have the connections that promise me a security unknown to those in the ghetto. And were all of the above taken away, I would still have a lifelong sense of entitlement to fall back on, far stronger than any entitlement program a government has ever conceived. I would have the secure psychological background of a childhood valued by parents, of trust in stable relationships, of confidence that I was able to handle whatever came to me in life. No matter what happens to me in the future, I will never share the experience of growing up poor and powerless within the abusive environment of the inner city.

If, by some perverse miracle, I managed to "join" the poor, I could never escape the fact of having chosen to. I would always be aware that, to become poor, I had purposefully relinquished the security that no poor person in his or her right mind would think me anything but crazy for giving away. I can never experience the essence of poverty: being trapped, without choice, in abominable conditions beyond my control. Mother Teresa's sisters take a vow of poverty so uncompromising that they may not even taste the delicacies at a reception given in their honor, but they *have* the reception and the abiding knowledge of having given their lives direction.

I live on the mainland of our society. No matter what route I choose, what decisions I make, I will always have a secure route back. The men downstairs live on an island, separated from me by waters deep and unbridgeable. Except through the distorted images of television, most of them hardly know what the mainland looks like. They might not recognize it if they happened on it by chance.

I am not complaining. The poverty of inner-city Washington is not to be sought. The spiritual discipline of "voluntary poverty" has nothing in common with the oppression and despair of the ghetto. There is nothing beautiful or romantic in frostbitten toes or minds destroyed by alcohol, in lives crushed by the weight of indifferent history and cultural negligence. The poverty of the inner city is evil, and we betray those caught in its web by romanticizing it or imagining that we—by divesting ourselves of some bits of our privilege—can choose to enter it. The landscape of poverty is inaccessible to most of us. We can barely imagine the scenery.

But neither is it possible to live as a privileged person within the world of the very poor without undergoing changes. We simply had not yet become aware of what they would be.

Chapter 5

Body Counts

The poor in our cities suffer a neglect and oppression that is unimaginable to the rest of us. Structures and institutions have been created that keep "us" separated from "them." Until recently, we of the middle class could avoid even seeing those who were very poor. Drive as a tourist through Washington today and you see a beautiful capital city of cherry blossoms and azaleas, monuments and parks, government buildings and high-priced, center-city shopping malls. As you travel around its main streets, the city looks predominantly white and affluent. You would hardly guess that the population is, in fact, seventy percent black, or that two miles from the White House is a ward where the infant mortality rate is higher than in many Third World countries. If—as a tourist—you travel by public transportation, gleaming subway cars will pull you smoothly into architecturally stunning stations. You will probably not notice that there are few stations in the poorer sections of town, or that the layout of the subway system best suits middle-class commuters from the suburbs, effectively excluding inner-city residents going from one place to another in their own city. It is on the buses, which wind through the city and turn a crosstown trip into a two-hour ordeal, that the poor do their traveling.

Poverty has both spread and deepened within our country during the last decade. Today you may see homeless men

78

and women sleeping on the steam grates near the National Mall or mothers panhandling with their children on Connecticut Avenue. You can read about the hopelessness of the ghetto's drug culture in Sunday's *Washington Post*. You may be accosted by beggars—both self-effacing and aggressive—in the wealthy enclave of Georgetown. But, even if poverty in our nation's capital has become more visible, you, as a visitor, will have little sense of the density of that poverty, little sense that you are viewing an oppressed people, little sense of the structures that guarantee that the poor will, by and large, remain poor.

No one knows how many homeless people there are in the United States. Within the city of Washington alone estimates vary, but most put the number at around 10,000—almost two percent of the population—and Washington seems quite representative of American cities. In 1990, government-supported and private shelters had about 2,500 beds available in Washington every night, but there were many people who did not sleep in the shelters. Henry Martin, one of my patients at Christ House, tells me that he and many of his friends prefer to sleep on the streets because the shelters are too dangerous; Rochelle Tippett and her baby shuttled for months from relative to relative, friend to friend, without stable housing. None of these homeless people takes up a shelter bed.

Efforts to count the homeless have all proved flawed. During the 1990 United States Census determined efforts were made, but the shifting, unstable nature of homeless people's living situations rendered the results questionable at best. Census officials actually attempted, on a particular night, to "cordon off" relatively small sections of some cities, search every abandoned building or hidden corner, and then extrapolate from their findings. In addition to the expected difficulties in finding the homeless, however, efforts were hampered by people who could not be—or didn't want to be—counted. Once, while traveling with the Health Care for the Homeless Project mobile health van, I met

Alfonso Matthews at a bus stop outside Union Station. Although homeless for many years, Mr. Matthews dresses daily in a three-piece suit and sits all day at the bus stop, indistinguishable from other government office workers waiting for buses. Later the same day I visited Harry Muldoon in an outdoor stairwell of the fashionable duplex on Capitol Hill where the owner allows him to sleep. How could any census taker record either of these men, or so many others whose homeless lives, by design and necessity, are hidden?

Disputes over the homeless body count have become a significant political issue. Many types of federal assistance are doled out on a per-person basis, so urban political representatives, eager for an increased share, argue that the urban homeless population has been drastically undercounted. Rural political representatives argue the opposite. Leaders of the Community for Christian Non-Violence refused to allow census officials into their large shelter in downtown Washington because they did not want to legitimize an enumeration that they believed would grossly underestimate the true homeless population. Under these complex circumstances, "definitive" body counts are impossible.

What is clear is that nationally, as in Washington, the problem of homelessness has been growing for several decades, slowly in the sixties and seventies and exponentially in the eighties and nineties. In 1987 alone, most American cities reported one-year increases in homelessness that were between fifteen and fifty percent.[4]

The surge in homelessness began with wholesale "deinstitutionalization." In the 1950s, the plight of the mentally ill, warehoused in large institutions, became news just as the first effective psychiatric medications were being developed. Experts believed that if patients were placed on those medications *and* if group housing, community mental health centers, residences for short-term psychiatric intervention, and ready access to hospitalization were provided, a large percentage of the institutionalized mentally ill could be cared for within the community, at a fraction of the previous cost.

The deinstitutionalization of the mentally ill became a bandwagon almost everyone could hop on: a humane, effective, and cheap solution to an ugly problem. Over the next decade, hundreds of thousands of patients were released from state hospitals onto the streets. As might have been predicted, however, the support systems upon which the process was predicated seldom materialized. Unable to care for themselves, large numbers of the mentally ill became the first victims of the present homelessness crisis. During the 1950s, for instance, the population at St. Elizabeth's, the only public psychiatric hospital in the Washington area, was over 5,000. By the mid-eighties, only 950 patients were still resident there. In contrast, a 1985 study of shelter residents in Washington estimated[5] that 1,200 homeless schizophrenics lived outdoors or in the shelters, making the streets the primary public "facility" for those suffering from this most disabling condition. And of all the office hours of all the 3,100 psychiatrists registered in the metropolitan area, "only twenty-five hours a week"— total—"were available for the homeless mentally ill, eight hours . . . paid for by the District's Mental Health Services Administration and seventeen hours . . . volunteered by various psychiatrists."[6]

The first shelters were small and makeshift, often church-run, and intended for the mentally ill, who are now a minority of the homeless. In spaces used by day for children's day-care centers or worship or Sunday school, beds were set up at night for five to fifteen men or women. Perhaps a meal was provided. Volunteers supervised. Soon these shelters were turning away far more than they could accommodate. Next to come were the larger, publicly funded shelters, usually single-sex, operated frequently out of old, unused schools or city buildings. In Washington, even trailers were hauled onto empty parcels of public property for use as shelters.

The typical profile of residents of these early shelters for

individuals (as opposed to families) showed high percent-
ages of mental illness and substance abuse, along with significant physical health problems. It was estimated, for
instance, that fifty-eight percent of the women and thirty-
three percent of the men who stayed in Washington's shelters in 1985 were schizophrenic.[7] Forty percent of the men
were also diagnosed as alcoholics. In a later Baltimore
study, ninety-one percent of homeless people surveyed had
at least one serious ("Axis I") psychiatric disorder.[8] These
mental health statistics translated into regular, random
violence—the results of which I frequently saw in my
office—as the emotional turmoil of lives without access to
care, much less psychiatric care, was acted out.
    Over the course of the eighties, the demographics of the
homeless population changed radically. There was no
longer a "typical" shelter resident. Shelters were still
crowded with skid-row derelicts and the severely mentally
ill, but now these were joined by young men whose full-
time salary wasn't enough to cover rent, older women separated from husband and family and unable to find work,
middle-aged men whose jobs had disappeared from the
economy—and steadily increasing numbers of young
women and their children. To a large extent, this change
was the result of a sharp decline in low-income housing.
During the 1960s and 1970s, new public housing, however
inadequate, was at least being built. As late as 1980, construction of 183,000 low-income housing units began across
the country during the calendar year, sponsored by the U.S.
Department of Housing and Urban Development (HUD).
But the Reagan administration slashed the federal housing
budget from $30 billion in 1980 to $7 billion by 1985.[9] As
was evident in our neighborhood, new construction all but
stopped. By 1985 new HUD housing starts had dropped almost ninety-five percent, to 9,700 units under construction.[10] This not only means that there is little affordable
housing for the poor at present, but that no more is coming.
Even were we to commit ourselves today as a nation to a
crash program to provide adequate housing for the poor, it

would—because construction takes so long—be years before those appropriations were translated into homes. In Washington, in 1992, there were over 11,000 families on the waiting list for public housing. Fifty-year-old Miriam Tesfaye, her daughter, and two grandchildren were finally notified that they would receive public housing ten *years* after having put their names on the list; the *average* time a family spends on the waiting list is five and a half years. Yet budgetary constraints and inefficiencies within the responsible city departments mean that, of the roughly 11,000 units of public housing of any kind in the city of Washington, over 2,000 lie vacant and in disrepair.

Bob Mayer, a former resident of Christ House, searched for more than six months before finding a single room in a decent boardinghouse for under $300 a month. The average single-bedroom apartment, even in the worst sections of town, rents for $650 a month, approximately the *entire* take-home pay of an unskilled worker at one of the fast-food restaurants like McDonald's in Adams-Morgan. A federal standard established during the 1980s considers housing to be "affordable" if a person or family spends less than thirty percent of income on it; but in the District of Columbia—as in many other American metropolitan areas—more than three in four poor families pay more than that, and one out of every four pays more than seventy-five percent of their entire income just for the roof over their heads.[11] In Washington, housing costs alone exceed the entire grant for families receiving assistance under Aid to Families with Dependent Children (AFDC).

People double- and triple-up with relatives and friends, so that it is not unusual to find five or even ten people living in one-bedroom apartments in our neighborhood. Young Raoul Martinez, who took the bus to elementary school with my son, Kai, lived with *twenty* other relatives in a single-family row house down the street. According to a special District of Columbia study, an estimated 31,600 families live in doubled-up households, accounting for 126,000 household residents—over twenty percent of the city's total population.[12] When, for any reason, such an arrangement fails, a family is likely to find itself out on the street or at one of the city's family shelters. In addition, much privately owned rental housing previously available to people with low incomes has been converted over the last decade into condominiums for the affluent. The poor are not in the streets by mistake. It is the only place left.

Occasionally my work took me to the large shelter on Second and D Streets in downtown Washington, only a few blocks from the Capitol. Because so little else was available, the Community for Creative Non-Violence had commandeered this abandoned and decaying city property in the early 1980s, declared it a shelter for homeless men and women, and opened the doors to anyone who wanted to sleep there. Most Washington shelters or other institutions serving the poor and homeless find themselves—because of limited budgets—in the city's hidden corners or on its out-of-the-way streets, but CCNV's Mitch Snyder, by simply invading a very desirable, vacant piece of real estate in the middle of federal Washington, created such political visibility that ultimately CCNV was not only allowed to remain but given substantial city and federal assistance. "Officially," 800 homeless persons stayed there during the colder months, although on the coldest winter nights, occupancy went as high as 1,400.

One morning Janelle asked me to substitute for her during her "office hours" at the shelter. I drove south from Belmont Street, down Fourteenth Street (known for years after 1968 as the "riot corridor"), beside burned-out and broken-down buildings, past prostitutes finishing their night shifts. As soon as I crossed Massachusetts Avenue, however, I found myself in a bustling, modern commercial city. Turning east, I was soon surrounded by imposing government buildings. Here, in the center of "official Washington," stood the decaying former campus of Federal City College.

As I stepped into the central hallway, the first thing I saw was the morning's breakfast, collected from several food stores the night before—hundreds of "day-old" hard rolls that had spilled from garbage bags onto the floor. But what struck me most forcefully was the pervasive smell of urine and feces.

I had not been in the building before, so a CCNV staff member gave me a brief tour. We walked through the "living quarters"—filthy rooms in which cots lay haphazardly, separated only by several feet of empty space. Grimy blankets lay rumpled on the cots, and cockroaches crawled everywhere. In many rooms, much of the ceiling had fallen, and in some the old plaster lay pushed into corners. The remains of rotting plasterboard, unusable wiring and ducting, and the floorboards of the room above were all that separated us from those living on the next floor. The stench from the men's restroom was overpowering. I could hardly believe that people used such facilities, and it was all I could do to force myself momentarily inside to look. Everywhere were signs of destruction: holes punched in walls, missing lights, broken windows.

Sister Lenora showed me the "health station" where she, Janelle, and a receptionist worked. The examining rooms were just parts of the hallway blocked off with low screens, but the patients seemed to have given up on the possibility of privacy long ago. There was no running water near the health station, so Lenora carried water in for washing and heated it on a burner—"just as we used to do when I was working in Thailand," she told me. Outside the window was a small courtyard piled perhaps a foot deep with trash, which rained continually from upper-floor windows. The only escape, in case of fire, would be through the huge building's two working exit doors, both of which were locked each night once the residents went to sleep.

Why would more than 800 men and women live together in this rat-infested shelter? Why would people *want* to live there? Presumably for the same reason that the CCNV, then with no money and little power, chose to keep it open: It was better than any other option they had.

Federal City Shelter has since been remodeled, but only because in 1984 Mitch Snyder and other members of the CCNV community went on a hunger strike that brought them near death and forced then-President Reagan—on the eve of the presidential election—to allocate $5 million for renovation. The degrading conditions I saw there have been corrected, but several other of the larger, publicly supported shelters in the city, like those in the old Blair and Pierce Schools in northeast Washington, still remind me of the CCNV warehouse. Smaller shelters, frequently church basements turned into overnight living accommodations, provide clean and relatively safe surroundings, but many close for the warmer months of the year. With the exception of CCNV's shelter at Second and D Streets, all of the larger and most of the smaller men's shelters close during the day, forcing their residents onto the streets from seven in the morning until seven at night. For most, the evening return is on a first-come, first-served basis. Women's shelters are generally not as large and allow residents a guaranteed return in the evening; a few have day programs, or at least allow the women to stay in during the day.

The city also has direct operational responsibility for a number of shelters designated specifically for families. Most of these families consist of only one parent, usually the mother, and several small children. In the mid-1980s, when the population of homeless families exploded and the fifty-two-family capacity of the Pitts Hotel no longer sufficed, the city began to rent rooms (and often entire motels) at a cost of about $2,500 per family per month, appropriately titling these widely dispersed motels "the open market." "Open-market families" lived overnight at the motels but—in some cases because the rooms were also rented out "by the hour" during the day, in other cases because the motel keepers didn't want permanent residents—the mothers (or, more rarely, fathers) and their children had to leave every morning, often taking all their belongings with them, sometimes meeting the "daytime renters" and their customers coming in or out. The Pitts Hotel remained the only site where meals and social services were provided. The young parents of these homeless families were, moreover, required by the city to spend their daytime hours actively seeking work and housing. It was all most could do, however, to traipse back and forth between the various checkpoints, much less keep their children in school, look for work, and search out an apartment.

In the spring of 1990, the City Council passed regulations that limited the amount of time individuals could stay in shelters and barred repeated use, effectively gutting a previously passed general referendum guaranteeing shelter to the homeless. Activists managed to place another, similar initiative on the ballot that fall, but—signaling a changing national mood—the electorate voted it down. Subsequent regulations similarly limited shelter options even for families. In 1991 and 1992, citing budgetary constraints and "empty beds," the District of Columbia began closing some of the public shelters, further reducing the number of beds available for the expanding homeless population. In 1993, the District was sued for having violated the rules that required cities accepting federal money for family shelter to guarantee access for all families. Rather than spend the extra $5 million from its own budget to meet those regulations, the city turned down over $10 million in federal assistance.

If the homeless are the most visible and dramatic representatives of "the Poor," they are only a small fraction of the group they represent. In the city of Washington, 17.4 percent of people live in households with incomes below the poverty line. Whites, who make up approximately thirty percent of the population, total only five percent of those living in poverty. In the predominantly white Third Ward, only three percent of families live in poverty; while in the almost exclusively black Seventh and

Eighth Wards, over twenty percent have incomes below the poverty level.°

Various forms of government assistance keep some people from falling below the poverty line, but the vast majority of these are the elderly receiving Social Security. The usual "welfare" benefits available to nonelderly poor people are so meager as to keep them mired in their difficulties. The primary form of assistance to families, Aid to Families with Dependent Children (AFDC), for instance, provides in 1993 a monthly income of $480 to a family of four—$633 below the poverty line. Public Assistance, the usual form of help for single individuals, is $260 monthly—$407 below the poverty line. These levels of financial aid are not adjusted for inflation (as is, for example, Social Security, which also benefits the nonpoor). The support they offer in real dollars, therefore, falls every year. If that weren't enough, the actual dollar amount of AFDC was cut in 1991; a family of three, which up until then received $428 a month, now receives $409.

The public education system further contributes to keeping the poor poor. Children of poverty normally attend third-rate public schools, where a successful day for a teacher may well consist of simply maintaining discipline. A member of our church who lived in the neighborhood, Georgia Murphy, opened her home to nine-year-old Melanie for what turned out to be a five-year respite from her father's violence. The girl, not surprisingly, had done poorly in school and had been kept behind her class. Geor-

° The federal "poverty level" itself underestimates what most of us would consider poverty. In the 1960s, the Federal Office of Economic Activity first defined the poverty level, arbitrarily, as three times what it would cost a family to buy the most basic food. This food budget itself derived from a Department of Agriculture "low-cost budget" that assumed the homemaker to be a careful shopper, a skillful cook, and a good manager; there was no provision for eating out or having guests. In other words, people living below the poverty level (who often pay over half their income for rent) cannot eat adequately even if they spend a third of their income on food, even assuming that the homemaker has all the stipulated skills (not infrequently lacking among people who have been reared amid the chaos of urban poverty).

gia knew that Melanie was bright and quite capable of doing grade-level work; when Georgia visited the school in an effort to intervene, however, she discovered that *all* of the children who had been kept behind from *any grade* went to class together in one large room, a sort of "one-room schoolhouse" for those in trouble. Georgia inquired about the curriculum so that she could help with Melanie's homework; the teacher informed her straightforwardly that there *was* no curriculum—the teacher had all she could do to keep order in the classroom, and there was certainly no time to teach six different class levels. For all practical purposes, there was no academic learning going on at all! After several further attempts at intervention, Georgia's only recourse was to move Melanie to another school where actual instruction would be available.

In Washington, as elsewhere, middle- and upper-class families either move to the suburbs (neighboring Montgomery County in Maryland and Fairfax County in Virginia have some of the best public schools in the country) or place their children in private schools. Even among the poor, the most resourceful parents can—like Georgia—take advantage of the city's policy of "open enrollment," which allows the most persistent to enroll their children in the better public schools outside their home district. Consequently, few of these parents remain involved in supporting, pressuring, or reforming their local schools.

The all-too-familiar result is that most of the city's black schoolchildren are ghettoized into a separate educational system. (Only 2.3 percent of public-high-school students, for instance, are white, and almost all of these attend one high school in the affluent upper Northwest neighborhood.) These schools for the poor—where the drop-out rate is the highest in the nation—must use a disproportionate amount of their budgets to contend with the effects of homelessness, hunger, and violence (both in the streets and within the home), to deal with the physical and emotional effects of poverty before they can even begin the day's education.[13] While salaries may be adequate, the best teachers leave these schools in discouragement or frustration after a few years because they rarely manage to get through the morass of other issues to do what they have been prepared to do— teach.

What do the ghetto's young people have to look forward to when they leave school and enter the workforce? Minimum-wage jobs, often in service industries, are generally available to those with little education, but jobs on which one can live independently, much less support a family, are scarce, partly because the minimum wage has not kept pace with inflation. In 1950, when federal minimum-wage standards were first established, the minimum wage was fifty-four percent of the average earnings of a production worker in manufacturing; by 1990 the minimum wage had dropped to thirty-five percent of that average production worker's wage, a relative loss of over one third. As a result, the earnings of a mother with two children, working *full-time, year-round* for the minimum wage, fell twenty-three percent below the poverty line.[14]

A good worker in the service sector, where most new jobs are to be found in Washington, might earn five dollars an hour (about $700 a month) take-home pay—slightly more than the average cost of a month's rent for a one-bedroom apartment in the District of Columbia. If a young family also wanted to buy health insurance (rarely provided in low-paying jobs), almost half of a second service-industry salary would be necessary. So even with two parents working full-time, a family might then have only $400 a month left for food, clothing, heat and light, child care, transportation, telephone, and perhaps something for entertainment. And I know very few families on Belmont Street with two parents, to say nothing of their both holding jobs. Community leaders estimate that over half the young men in our community are unemployed. On every side the poor are hemmed in, trapped into pockets of poverty.

Despite the institutionalized neglect poor people suffer in the areas of housing, public assistance, education, and employment, what shocked me most as a physician was the limited health care available to them. Having worked in Minnesota, where I knew of no doctor who turned away poor people because of their inability to pay, and having taken a year's sabbatical in Marja's homeland of Finland, where everyone is assured of high-quality health care, I was startled by Louise Flowers's statement that her private physician had refused her care because she could no longer afford to pay for it. In fact, I didn't really believe she was telling me the truth. Hearing so many similar stories from other patients, however, I conceived a simple, informal study of local private physicians.

Rita Branham—the young woman who had lived in the abandoned and decaying Community of Hope building before it was purchased, and who was now working with me as a medical assistant—volunteered to telephone fifty primary-care doctors (family practitioners, obstetricians, and pediatricians) in the District of Columbia to try to make an appointment. As a longtime resident of the Belmont Street neighborhood, she knew well the realities of poverty and also spoke the local dialect. (One clue to the depth of segregation in Washington is the persistence of a ghetto dialect that can be virtually unintelligible to the speaker of standard English. Although the dialect is certainly an important cultural heritage, the inability of most inner-city residents to speak standard English both represents and contributes significantly to the separation of the poor black person from the mainstream of society. Rita is herself "bilingual," speaking standard English well, yet many of the people she grew up with are not—further evidence that they live, quite literally, in another world.)

I asked Rita to try to make an appointment with each of the fifty physicians as if she were still indigent and could not afford to pay full price at the time of the visit. Only one out of ten physician's receptionists would give her an appointment; the others had *no* provision either for reducing the doctor's fees based on her income level or even for allowing her to pay over time. A middle-class person down on her luck who nevertheless knew how to negotiate the system might be able to find that one physician in ten, or be able to talk her way into one of the other nine offices. But a poor person without insurance or a hundred dollars cash in hand could not see a private doctor.

Rita then informed those who wouldn't give her an appointment that she had Medicaid. Over half of the remaining doctors' offices still refused to give her an appointment. What Medicaid will pay is declining relative to what physicians charge; consequently, more and more doctors are refusing to treat patients who are on Medicaid. Recently, despite multiple phone calls, we could not find a single private obstetrician in the city who would accept a Medicaid patient of ours.

Medicaid is federally funded, but because each state administers its own program, eligibility criteria vary. In states like New York, the program is widely available to the poor, but reimbursement is so low that it doesn't even cover the doctor's overhead costs. In other jurisdictions, such as the District of Columbia, Medicaid pays enough to allow a physician at least to cover expenses, but it is only accessible to a minority of the poor. To receive Medicaid in the District of Columbia, one has to be both poor *and* the single parent of small children or poor *and* completely disabled according to rigid Social Security Administration criteria. Suggs, penniless and sick as he was, did not qualify for Medicaid; it took us over four years to get Medicaid for John Turnell, even though he obviously qualified. It's not just inadequate reimbursements and increased paperwork, however, that prompt doctors to refuse Medicaid patients; doctors whom I have questioned directly often cite the fear that poor patients will drive away their other clients. Whatever reason is offered, the effect is the same: A poor person can't even get in the door of most doctors' offices.

In all other developed nations except South Africa—whose status as a developed nation may be in question—some form of national health insurance provides basic access to health care for all citizens regardless of their ability to pay. In the United States, only thirty-one percent of people with incomes below the poverty level qualify for Medicaid.[15] And of those who would qualify, many are not on the rolls, either because the regulations have been applied inconsistently or because the application process is so daunting as to discourage one's trying. The vast majority of poor adults whom I see as patients (District *children*, fortunately, are often enrolled in Medicaid) have no medical coverage—not even for doctors' visits.

In the past few years, the situation has become worse. Teaching hospitals' clinics, staffed by resident physicians-in-training and supervised by attending physicians, have traditionally been an entry point for the poor into the health care system. But by 1990, every private hospital in Washington except Children's Hospital had stopped accepting uninsured, indigent patients into these clinics. In 1992 I was told by several physicians at a large, prestigious private hospital that they were being pressured by the administration to limit even the number of Medicaid patients accepted into their clinics.

Like everybody else, I hope that the current debate over universal health care and the proposals put forward by the Clinton administration will yield adequate health coverage for all. And there's an argument to be made that any change in the health care provisions for the poor would have to be an improvement. Political realities appear to be such, however, that the administration's proposals are likely to have little positive impact on the care available to the poor. Because of intense opposition from the insurance industry and much of the medical establishment, the president's commission never seriously considered a single-payer national health insurance plan—the only option capable of generating the revenue to cover the almost 40 million currently uninsured Americans without raising overall costs.[16] In the absence of such a plan, it's hard to see where the funding could possibly come from to cover the uninsured. And as of this writing—as might have been predicted—the dates for extending coverage to various uncovered groups are being pushed off into what will probably be an indefinite future. Further, the current proposals could make things *worse* for certain groups of poor people. If, as suggested, Medicaid enrollees are shifted out of a public program and enrolled in private health maintenance organizations with the proposed co-payments, the cost to a poor family even for services covered by the program could consume more than twenty-five percent of family income.[17] And services covered by the basic benefit package will, in Washington at least, be less than Medicaid currently offers.

But funding is not the only issue. Washington, like any large American city, boasts a set of institutions already funded whose specific task it is to care for the abandoned of our society. From D.C. General Hospital to child protective services, from general public assistance to tuberculosis clinics, the range of services is broad and the number of people employed immense. Public ambulatory care clinics provide well-child care (including immunizations), prenatal care, and regular preventive care for adults. Three mental health clinics see 4,300 patients yearly. The detoxification unit at D.C. General Hospital will take anyone, regardless of ability to pay, and two other detox units at private hospitals accept Medicaid patients.

Given the numbers, there should be little problem with access to these services, and those critics who would discount the value of social programs and blame the poor for their own poverty can point to a seeming overabundance of publicly financed assistance. But there is a surprising variety of obstacles.

One morning we tried to make an appointment at a public ambulatory care clinic for a patient we could not accommodate. From nine o'clock to ten, no one there answered the phone. From ten to eleven, we were told that "the person in charge of appointments is out"; then no answer again until "the person in charge of appointments is at lunch," and so on. When we finally made contact that afternoon, it turned out there was no time set aside that day or the next for patients without long-standing appointments: A person needing immediate attention simply couldn't get into the clinic. As I tried to coordinate medical care for very poor people, I repeatedly came up against institutions that had set up so many barriers that they were, for all practical purposes, inaccessible to the very people they were founded to serve.

These ambulatory care clinics—like D.C. General Hospital, the city's child protective services, mental health clinics, and other public institutions—have been caught between declining budgets and an increasing caseload. More and more, as caregivers are overwhelmed by the problems they face, the result has been that patients slip through the cracks; and when one is already at the bottom of society, to "slip through the cracks" is to land somewhere unimaginable to the rest of us.

Mr. Connor was a homeless man living from shelter to shelter. Because of severe frostbite, his left leg had previously been amputated just above the knee. In my eight years as a doctor in the northern Minnesota wilderness, a frequent destination for winter campers, I only once saw frostbite severe enough to require amputation, and then only of several toes. Frostbite may result from the occasional mountaineering accident but is otherwise a rare injury—except among those homeless in our cities who, for whatever reason, must spend all day and even all night outside. For them, frostbite is a common affliction, and amputation of fingers, toes, feet, and legs is often a necessity.

One February night, Mr. Connor was brought by ambulance to the emergency room of D.C. General, suffering from frostbite in his remaining leg. In the emergency room he was seen and evaluated by a physician who instructed him to elevate the leg, keep it clean, and return to an appropriate D.C. General clinic in several days to have the wounds cared for. The emergency room physician (without first determining whether there would even be a bed available for Mr. Connor) then arranged for him to be transported back to the door of the overnight shelter at which he had been staying. But Mr. Connor had spent the evening in the emergency room. It was now past ten o'clock, and the beds in the shelter had already been allotted. Had a compassionate shelter supervisor not intervened and arranged to transfer him to Christ House, Mr. Connor would have had to spend another night in below-freezing weather on the street. Considering his condition, he might well have died. When Mr. Connor arrived, we found an emaciated, helpless man, his one foot oozing and gangrenous. Above the foot were two blisters from frostbite, each about six inches by three inches in size. When we turned him over to undress and bathe him, we discovered three large pressure sores, one more than an inch deep, over his tailbone and buttocks, the result of sitting in one position for hours at a time in his wheelchair, which had somewhere along the way lost its cushioning. Mr. Connor was a very sick man.

Fortunately we were able to arrange immediate admission to a private hospital, but the frostbitten leg was already badly infected, and the infection had spread to his bloodstream. Even with the best in-hospital care, the remaining leg had to be amputated less than forty-eight hours later. Mr. Connor stayed in the intensive care unit for many days, fighting against a life-threatening infection of the blood. Except for the fact that he survived his initial hospitalization, I do not know what happened to Mr. Connor. I cannot imagine that he would have been discharged back to the streets in his condition—even in Washington. Maybe he was fortunate enough to get a spot in a nursing home.

It is possible, of course, that the resident who sent Mr. Connor back into the night was a physician-in-training at D.C. General who simply did not know what he or she was looking at. It is possible that Mr. Connor was not able to articulate his complaint very well and was never undressed and examined thoroughly. But I have seen too many poor people discharged from crowded public emergency rooms—sometimes with feet black from gangrene, other times with obvious symptoms of cancer or serious complications of AIDS. I have seen too many Mr. Connors, in effect, to believe that their inadequate treatment is simply the luck of the draw. If a middle-class person with Mr. Connor's level of illness had come to any emergency room in the city, he or she would have been admitted immediately and without question. The public hospitals provide to the poor a level of treatment the rest of us would find absolutely unacceptable.

The obstacles, even to such care as this, are manifold. In cases such as Medicaid, treatment is restricted to a particular category of people, leaving large numbers of equally needy people totally without access. In other cases, such as the inpatient alcohol and drug rehabilitation program at Karrick Hall, all are eligible and the institution performs remarkably with excellent results—but the need far outstrips the resources. Karrick Hall, for instance, is the only inpatient rehabilitation program in the District of Columbia; the length of its waiting list varies but is now seven months.

In other institutions and departments, all needy persons are eligible for services, but human resources are stretched so thin that no one gets adequate attention. Social workers at Child Protective Services, for instance, have to manage caseloads of between sixty and one hundred or more—an impossible task.

In still other instances the service providers are burned out and need help themselves: They have become so numbed to the suffering around them that they can no longer do their jobs with compassion or enthusiasm.

About a year after my arrival in Washington, I was invited to participate in a series of meetings regarding the care of indigent and homeless tuberculosis patients. Representatives from area hospitals, from the city's public health department, and from other health organizations came together with private physicians to share information and make recommendations to the city on how to slow the spread of tuberculosis among the homeless and the poor generally. As a relative newcomer to Washington, I was proud to be asked, and I nurtured a secret hope that my experiences on the "front lines" might command enough respect to give my opinions weight. Janelle's patient Mr. Solten, who had received such poor care at the hands of "the System," was fresh in my mind; surely anyone could see that the system *must* function better than this! I hoped my righteous indignation would translate into specific recommendations for change.

I brought with me a list of patients who, like Mr. Solten, had "fallen through the cracks" of the public system mandated to deal with tuberculosis. I mentioned Michael Farley, who had died of tuberculosis and its complications two weeks previously at D.C. General. Wilbur Morris, the administrator of Area C Chest Clinic and an assistant, Murine Chostek, looked at each other as I mentioned Mr. Farley's name . . . and they laughed! "Oh, yes, we know about Michael Farley. He was a real old-time TB patient. He was always real difficult to keep track of."

The laughter knocked me off balance. "We think he was probably homeless," I said, trying to get the discussion back on track.

"No, I don't think so," Mr. Morris replied. "He lived with his brother. He might have become homeless recently, I don't know about that, but he used to live with his brother. We just never could keep track of him. I *knew* he was going to die from it."

Area C was responsible for providing outpatient treatment to anyone (including the homeless) with tuberculosis who could not obtain private medical attention. If such patients wouldn't come in, Mr. Morris and his staff were supposed to find them wherever they were and administer their medications. If a patient refused altogether, Mr. Morris had the authority to initiate legal proceedings to confine him or her until cured. What did their laughter mean? Why didn't the others in the room seem offended by it?

A few minutes later the case of a Mr. Collins arose. Mr. Collins was a patient with active tuberculosis who had stayed for a time at Adams House. A nurse from Area C stopped by three times a week to give him his antibiotics.

After Mr. Collins found a private room in a Community Residence Facility (CRF), a publicly funded group home, however, the visits from Area C had for some reason stopped, and his disease had recurred. When his name came into the discussion, Mr. Morris and Ms. Chostek once again glanced knowingly at each other and laughed as if the fact that he was untreated were a joke between them. "Oh, Bobby Collins," said Ms. Chostek. "He's another one. We haven't been able to get hold of him to give him his treatment. You just can't keep track of some of these people." "You mean you don't know where he is?" someone asked.

"Oh, Bobby was staying at some CRF, but he moved out and we couldn't find him. Besides, he leaves early in the morning and comes back late at night. He was never there when we came by." Once again, the knowing laugh.

(Later, I asked Sister Lenora about Mr. Collins. She knew him well. She immediately called Adams House and ascertained within minutes the address of the CRF at which he was currently staying. I mentioned that the public health people couldn't "get hold of" him. "Well, you do have to do a little detective work," she said. "I used to go by his place first thing in the morning to catch him. Sometimes I could even schedule a time to meet with him. If we asked him, I think he'd go back over to Adams House to get his medicines.")

Soon after, a third name came up, that of one James Mattley, a schizophrenic patient previously treated for tuberculosis and recently readmitted to one of the local hospitals with active TB. He was also well known to Area C. Again there were the chuckles and smiles. He had been treated several times, they said, but always dropped out of treatment. A hopeless case. (Later, doing the legwork ourselves, we found out that he had been hospitalized at St. Elizabeth's, the public psychiatric hospital, where—no thanks to Area C Chest Clinic—his tuberculosis was being appropriately treated.)

It was the laughter that upset me most. I had come prepared to point out the lack of care for persons seriously ill with tuberculosis, naïvely thinking that these officials did not know what was going on. I was totally unprepared to have the plight of these sick men and women treated as a joke. I was angry, but my colleagues' laughter effectively silenced me. I didn't know what to say. The others in the room sat impassively, either silenced like myself or—for one reason or another—unconcerned.

Only much later, when I began to experience some of the burnout associated with my work, was I able to reflect upon what had probably happened. I realized then that these public health officials were responsible for a number of patients whom they categorized—for whatever reason—as "hopeless," as patients "nobody could help." These professionals, who saw themselves as "helpers," protected themselves from the sting of self-recrimination by those knowing laughs that said, "Oh, he's one of *them*. We can't really do much." Deciding that a patient was beyond help made it easier to justify not trying very hard. If the men didn't fit into clinic schedules, if they were difficult to track down— well, what more could be done, after all?

Given the complicated set of economic, social, psychological, and health problems they presented, Mr. Solten, Mr. Farley, Mr. Collins, and Mr. Mattley *were* difficult cases to deal with. No matter how highly motivated Mr. Morris was, he would have had great difficulty coping with their needs. Undoubtedly too little money was available for Area C, and too few caseworkers, to offer the kind of individual attention for which Sister Lenora found the energy. Certainly homelessness, lack of education, poor nutrition, and untreated alcoholism were problems about which Mr. Morris could do little or nothing. Perhaps he simply did not have the resources, personal or institutional, to deal with the burnout of his staff—or in himself. Perhaps his derisive laughter was the only way he could handle the tragedy of it all.

That day, I had no such sympathy for Mr. Morris. It took me many more months to entertain the possibility that Mr.

Morris was not as heartless as he had appeared. Was it not likely that he had once been deeply concerned about the problems of poverty and injustice and their effect on the health of poor people? Otherwise why would he have taken on such a thankless job? But somewhere, sooner or later, his compassion had been overwhelmed and had withdrawn to where it was invisible, perhaps even to him. Then, no longer believing himself part of a solution, he had become just another part of the problem.

"Mr. Morris" is a species commonly found in any branch of public service. For all my understanding, I still frequently find myself angry with people like him and blame them for the suffering of my patients. It seems to me that it is precisely in those institutions charged with serving the poor that one finds the highest proportion of workers who are no longer responsive to the real needs of their clients. When the receptionist at the public health clinic desk no longer really cares whether you get an appointment with the doctor; when the doctor no longer has hope that you can get better; when the administrator no longer believes that one can run a clinic to truly serve the needs of the indigent, the ultimate result is another institution that encumbers the poor, another strand in the web that binds them so tightly to deprivation.

Chapter 6

FAMILY MATTERS

It is late evening, perhaps nine-thirty. Marja and I and our children have been at dinner with friends and are walking back to our apartment, enjoying a chance to chat together. We reach the street just behind Christ House. It is October, and the weather is still warm. Light from old-fashioned streetlamps casts a gentle glow on the tiny, neatly manicured lawns in front of row houses, and I think to myself, "I could almost like this city."

Suddenly, I'm aware of voices behind us, unintelligible growlings hurled in our direction. I wheel around to see a group of adolescent boys. A step in front of the others, no older than fifteen, stands the one who has spoken, looking levelly at me from perhaps ten feet away, pointing a pistol directly into my face.

"Drop your pack, mister!"

Every bit of me freezes. My mind flashes to the $200 in my wallet. I withdrew it from the automatic teller machine this afternoon and foolishly forgot to leave it at home. Although I always carry some cash (the only thing worse, I've been told, than a Washington mugger finding lots of money in your pocket is his finding none), I make it a rule not to walk around with more than twenty or thirty dollars. Things like this happen in our neighborhood.

I've had fantasies about how I would respond to such a situation, ranging from a deft kick at chest level, knocking

102

the gun from my assailant's hand, to a magnanimous offer to help a person so obviously in trouble. But this is the real thing, and I can't move. I can't even think. It's not that the money's so precious or that I'm stupid enough to challenge a punk with a gun. I'm simply frozen to the spot, unable to function.

There is more unintelligible jeering from the other boys in the group, and laughter. What are they high on? What's going on?

"I said drop your pack, mister!" There isn't a bit of emotion in the voice. I can see the softness of youth in his face, but somehow it doesn't register. A spring clicks as he cocks the trigger. I am looking straight into the barrel of a gun. He pulls the trigger. Click! He pulls it again. Click!

Suddenly, the boys break into shouts and hoots. As they run, laughing, down the street, I see in my mind's eye what I had looked at but not grasped before: The barrel into which I was gazing was solid. It was a toy!

I am still hardly able to move, paralyzed by shock. My legs are rubbery and I feel dizzy, exhausted, my heart furiously pounding. As first movement, then thought, and finally emotion return, I'm briefly grateful and then enraged. A basic sense of security snaps and is gone. Deep within I now *feel* my own vulnerability to the chaos of the city: physical vulnerability.

I had always known in some abstract way that I would be helpless against any person—adult or child—who grabbed a gun and decided to hold me up, but now I feel it as a palpable certainty. If the boys with the toy gun had stayed around a little longer, they would have gotten my backpack and probably the $200. At age fourteen, they were just playing a stupid and dangerous game. In a couple of years, it would no longer be make-believe.

When we first decided on Washington, I assumed we would live in the surrounding countryside or suburbs and that I would commute to the inner city. I couldn't imagine our children growing up in even the "best" parts of the city . . .

and we weren't headed for the best parts. But Marja believed that we needed to live in the midst of our work. We wanted our lives to be integrated, she reminded me; we wanted our work, our family life, our spiritual lives, our recreation to be part of a single fabric. Most important, we wanted our children to understand what we were doing with our lives, and why. Marja intuited that if we lived outside the city I would—as far as the children were concerned—be simply one more father commuting to his urban job. It would make only a marginal difference to them whether I provided medical services to the poor or shuffled papers in a government office. The children would suffer the consequences of my preoccupation with my work without experiencing the benefits of our life with the poor. Like all parents, I suppose, we wanted our children to accompany us on at least part of our journey.

But how could we subject them to the chaos of the inner city? How could we send them to those schools? Would twelve-year-old Laurel or nine-year-old Karin be safe on the sidewalks? Could four-year-old Kai find grass on which to play? To what risks were we exposing them? And these were only *our* questions: Who knew what theirs were or would be, what fears or expectations they would have?

Marja's and my vocation lay in the inner city, but was it fair to insist that the children follow us? We certainly did not want to coerce them into the more "simplified" life we were choosing, and we felt we had no right to insist that they make the same choices we were making. On the other hand, we were aware that no matter what our choices as parents, Marja and I would be pushing one kind of lifestyle or another. Rural Minnesota had imposed certain limitations on our children, too, as would the suburbs if we moved there. After much discussion and reflection, we decided that our living in the inner city would encourage them to consider justice, the suffering of the poor, and the dilemma of their affluence as they thought about the meaning of their lives—and ours.

We had been warned about the terrible state of public education in Washington. Would it be possible to find schools we considered adequate for our children? We sought out a couple—white, middle-class people like ourselves who had come to the city to be involved with the poor and had placed their children in the local public school—and spent an evening talking about education in the city. They believed deeply in the value of neighborhood public schools, they said. They had wanted their children to grow up without the subtle prejudices they themselves had developed about the poor and about people of color. But after their boys had spent two years in their neighborhood elementary school, these parents began to discover that the realities of class and privilege were not so easy to overcome. Their sons, who had grown up in a middle-class home and been exposed to considerable intellectual stimulation, stood academically so far above the rest of the students that they were having trouble relating to their classmates. They were being singled out, set apart. If anything, they were becoming *more* prejudiced, both by seeing themselves so far ahead of the other children and by feeling so isolated. Our friends eventually transferred their children to a racially and culturally mixed public school in upper Northwest, an affluent quarter of Washington several miles away where the boys found out—when confronted by a normally demanding educational environment—that they were not geniuses but average students.

It did not take us too much reflection to compromise our previous commitment to local, public school education. Enrollment in the Washington schools is open, and theoretically a student can attend any school in any district as long as space remains after the enrollment of all children from that district who want to attend. The better schools, of course, usually have long waiting lists for children from outside their districts. But because of school district gerrymandering—an attempt to bring children from our poorer neighborhood into wealthier upper Northwest Washington—our oldest daughter, Laurel, was already eligible for enrollment in Alice Deal Junior High School, a re-

putedly good public school about three miles away. We
made inquiries and discovered that our middle daughter,
Karin, then in fourth grade, could—because of an unusual
administrative coincidence—be admitted to John Eaton, a
public elementary school in upper Northwest, even though
the neighborhood school she would otherwise have attended, Bancroft Elementary, was just across the street. Because siblings were given precedence on the waiting list,
our son, Kai, then four, was eventually also accepted at
John Eaton. This seemed to us a reasonable compromise:
Deal and Eaton were both public schools, priding themselves on their racial and cultural diversity, and both
seemed to be providing solid educational experiences for
their students.

Some matters were not as easily resolved. Safety, for example. After we'd moved to Christ House, the children of
our neighborhood started getting hassled by a gang of young
boys who lived a few blocks away. A group of them—
apparently eyeing his bicycle—chased Kai, then eight years
old, down the street (he escaped by darting into the fire
station—a story he later told with some relish). Another
day they demanded money from him on his way back from
buying milk at the Safeway. After that, Kai refused to go
out alone for about six months. From our balcony one day
I watched this minigang of eight-to-twelve-year-olds in our
back alley as they circled around the tall, brawny parent of
a child whose bicycle they had stolen. The man had one of
the boys firmly by the arm, trying to force him to disclose
where he had hidden the bicycle. But the brazenness of the
other children startled me, for the rest of the group followed not ten yards away, throwing stones and taunting.
One part of me—educated through my experiences at the
clinic—looked upon the scene with the eye of a detached
professional: The children's behavior was symptomatic of
societal failure; an expression of their rage at their poverty
in a culture that labels poverty the deepest failure imaginable; an expression of their sense that there was little for
them to lose. But another part of me—the father of an

eight-year-old boy—was furious. I could well believe that Kai was helpless against them, and I supported his decision to stay off the streets. I felt anger, pain, and not a little guilt at his confinement. After several months the gang apparently disbanded; at least, they left our neighborhood, and Kai began playing outside once again.

My patients, too, occasionally reminded me of the dangers of living where we did and bringing our children into this inner city. One of the young men I admitted to Christ House had worked at Church's Fried Chicken, several blocks from us. He was walking home from work when four men accosted him, demanding money. He had none, and they—apparently believing he was about to use a gun (which he also didn't have)—shot him three times at point-blank range. Miraculously, he survived.

Virtually every one of my patients has had a close friend or relative killed or seriously injured. Bessie Wadders came into the office to ask for sleeping pills for a few nights because her son Delonzo had been shot and killed the day before; it is not an uncommon request at Community of Hope. Two weeks later, Madeline Keefe also came in needing sleeping pills: Her eighteen-year-old son Robert had just been arrested for killing Delonzo Wadders.

On a regular basis I take care of men and women who have been mugged in the neighborhood. Although as white, middle-class people living where we do, our family was in much less danger of attack than the poor black people living a few blocks away, one of our Christ House volunteers (also white and middle class) was dragged from a well-lighted street half a block from Christ House into an alley, attacked, and threatened with rape. A stranger, fortuitously passing by, scared the man off. Lynn Smith, the nursing assistant who works with me at the clinic, was caught in crossfire while walking to her neighborhood store with her children; she was seriously injured by a bullet to the neck and chest. A woman living three blocks away from us apparently refused to give money to someone who approached her at the entrance to her building; she was stabbed to death in front of her young children. A young man was gunned down in a drive-by shooting only two blocks from Christ House, where Kai found him moments later.

We are well aware that we are not secure.

At the same time, we live in middle-class comfort and order. Visitors' reactions as I guide them through Christ House reflect the paradox of our life. "I didn't expect it to look . . . uh . . . well . . . so nice," they stammer. "It's so new!" The building is spacious and airy, the kitchen large and fully equipped; an elevator moves us effortlessly between floors; two televisions, a VCR, and a stereo system are available for entertainment. On the second floor the men's bedrooms, while filled to capacity, are clean and attractive. It is sometimes hard to believe that these men moving quietly about are the same people one sees lying on benches and in the dark corners of the city.

When we climb the stairs and open the locked doors into the third- and fourth-floor hallways leading to our living areas, some visitors seem almost taken aback by "how nice it is." Since our living space remains off-limits to the men downstairs, the halls are quiet (unless the kids are home). Locked doors and coded elevators protect us and our families not only from the potentially psychotic or violent guest downstairs (in point of fact, such people have rarely been a risk), but also give us much greater protection against outside intruders than anyone else in the neighborhood enjoys. The fourth-floor chapel, with its beautiful tapestry, provides a place of stillness and peace unavailable, I would guess, in even the most luxurious apartment buildings. And the large third-floor community room becomes—when we need it—a rec room with Ping-Pong table and adjoining kitchen available for us, our guests, and volunteers.

The last stop on the tour, my family's private apartment—with its stereos, computers, variety of clothes, and well-stocked refrigerator—is little different from any middle-class apartment anywhere (even down to its controlled disarray). Each of our three children has a separate bedroom. When we moved into Christ House, friends of ours with interior decorating experience helped Laurel and Karin create tasteful individual rooms. Kai uses the hallway that runs from our apartment door down the length of the building as his back yard, creating in season a basketball court, soccer field, hockey rink, or football field. When the children want to talk with their suburban friends, there is a "children's phone" for their use. And the separate residential entrance at the side of the building allows my daughters to bring their school friends home without—if they choose—ever encountering a homeless person.

At the end of the tour, our guests' reactions vary widely. Even after seeing the place, some visitors still seem to view us as living the ghetto life of the poor. They can hardly imagine such "sacrifice" and are convinced that those of us who live and work here are a different breed, able somehow to endure almost unimaginable insecurity and deprivation. To others, however, our living conditions seem almost too luxurious, although politeness usually prevents them from articulating the question in their minds: How can Christ House in good conscience solicit donations from people struggling to make ends meet, while the staff lives so comfortably? And to still others—often those contemplating similar work for themselves—the relative comfort of our surroundings seems reassuring. I can imagine them saying to themselves: "Well, this isn't so bad. I could certainly see myself living here. Maybe this kind of work would be possible for us, too. If this is the 'sacrifice' people talk about, we can certainly manage it."

A similar phenomenon—this time in the area of salaries—occurs when I visit medical schools to talk about my experience as an inner-city doctor. Once in a while, during the discussion period after my speech—in which I usually mention the need for physicians to reduce their salaries to a more reasonable level—a student will ask the direct question: "Well, how much do *you* earn? What is your salary?" I am always a little uneasy with my answer. In 1993, a full-time physician's salary at Christ House is almost

$34,000, along with a rent-free apartment. When I mention the figure, however, I can sense the distinct reactions within the audience. A majority of the medical students automatically judge me among the religiously fanatic: "$34,000 and a little apartment! No way! That may be all right for him and his family but . . . well, let's be serious about this. I'm bothered by what's happening to the poor, too, but you can't expect doctors to carry all the burden!" These students see our lifestyle as highly self-sacrificing, strange, perhaps masochistic.

Others of these future physicians seem almost betrayed by my affluence. They expect, I suppose, a Mother Teresa or a Dorothy Day, living in poverty with the poor. And yet another part of the audience appears almost reassured: "$34,000 plus an apartment in the city! That's not so bad. That's more than my father makes. It's more than my husband and I have been living on for the past ten years; it's certainly nowhere near the poverty level I thought he was talking about. Perhaps I could consider doing something like this, too."

In choosing to live next to the poor, of course, we know that whatever insecurity, whatever "poverty" we experience is dwarfed by theirs.

Belinda is eighteen years old, the mother of two young children, and homeless. She is staying with her children up the street from Community of Hope at the Pitts Hotel. Belinda feels overwhelmed by the demands of being a single parent and frequently has only a tenuous grip on reality. Sometimes she's afraid she's possessed by the devil, afraid she'll injure her children. During one counseling session with Lois Wagner, Belinda volunteers that she used to dream of a better life, but that she doesn't dream anymore. Lois asks her what kinds of dreams she used to have. Gesturing to indicate the counseling room, simply furnished with a couch, two or three chairs, a stereo, and some pictures on the walls, Belinda replies, "Well, I certainly never dreamt I'd live in a beautiful house like this one."

Belinda has lost even the ability to imagine anything more than what I would consider substandard housing. When I, on the other hand, came to believe that the local schools would be damaging to my children, I had the power to get them out. When even the best public schools seemed inadequate, I knew that private school scholarships were always available for families like ours who have the knowledge and connections to find, apply for, and take advantage of them—which we did. (Both older girls eventually transferred to private schools in the Washington area.) It takes a middle-class perspective even to imagine that such alternatives exist. I take these internal resources for granted, but I can no more give away that sense of possibility than my patients can acquire it. Our family has chosen to simplify our lives and move closer to the poor, but the distance remains infinite and our gestures sometimes seem little more—even to us—than another middle-class luxury.

It is money, of course, that most obviously separates us from the poor. Living among thirty-four homeless men; walking among the panhandlers on Columbia Road; discovering that a patient did not take an important antibiotic because she could not afford the fifty-cent Medicaid co-payment (but was too embarrassed to tell me)—I am continually confronted by my own affluence and privilege, even in my work with the poor.

When I treat a patient who must spend more than half her income on rat-infested housing in a drug-ridden neighborhood; when I try unsuccessfully to arrange hospitalization for an individual with no access to adequate health care; when I see a five-year-old child stunted by poverty, basic questions confront me. In what sense do I *deserve* my wealth? If I possess these luxuries while they suffer in poverty, can there ever be community between me and my patients at Community of Hope? What happens to my sense of integrity when I live so comfortably while those with whom I would be friends remain—by accident of birth—homeless and marginalized? Many of my patients have been oppressed by the system that serves me very well. It is not always easy to return to the comfort of my home knowing that they are on the streets . . . especially when my home is a third-floor apartment just meters from where they may be sleeping.

How do my patients experience my affluence? Do they feel it creates a barrier between us? Are they resentful? Does it interfere with my doctoring? I don't know. I have been directly challenged on my relative wealth only once—by John Turnell, and then only when he was intoxicated. We in the middle-class community of helpers occasionally discuss the implications of our affluence for our work, and I suspect my patients discuss it among themselves. But we do not talk with one another about the disparities in our wealth. And that simple fact—that we never talk about what is, after all, one of the major differences between us—is stark evidence of the gulf that separates us.

Our work in the inner city has demanded some willingness to live more frugally. The thousands of individuals who support Christ House and Community of Hope by writing checks would be much less likely to donate their hard-earned dollars to pay me a $120,000 yearly salary. Our supporters quite properly expect us to live simply. In addition, our living so close to the overwhelming needs of the poor means that we are continually aware of the direct trade-off: At Christ House every dollar spent on salary is one dollar less for the needs of the men who live with us. Because the needs of the poor are so obvious and the trade-off so immediate, it seems simply wrong to pay ourselves more than we need to live in basic comfort.

But what is "basic comfort"? How does one decide on a proper standard of living? Clearly my salary is more than is necessary for the "basics" of food, clothing, and shelter: We have been willing to simplify our lives only so far. Brother Roger of the Taize religious community in France, which is committed to living in solidarity with the poor, recommends at least seven years for the transition from affluence to simplicity. No one need be ashamed about his place on such a journey, it seems to me, no matter how minimal the beginning steps may seem. Too many of us who are gradually discovering that there is a richness in voluntary simplification feel embarrassed to speak openly about our attempts because we know we have taken only small steps and don't want to expose ourselves to criticism. We are so troubled by the limits of our progress that we hesitate to speak of the journey at all, leaving others who would make a similar journey isolated and without models.

We must share our beginning steps with one another. If each of us has to invent the wheel all over again, our journeys become naïve, solitary, narrow. The experiences of each of us in moving closer to a just lifestyle are of value to others who want to do likewise.

There is, of course, considerable tension—and not a little contradiction—in our position. We cannot move into the world of the poor, but we are no longer quite at home in our own. Since it was most often our *children's* desires that had to be justified in light of the needs of those around us, it was the children who suffered most from these tensions and were most sensitive to the contradictions. They were also often most willing to bring them to their parents' attention.

At age thirteen, Laurel desperately wants braces for her teeth. Our dentist has recommended an orthodontist who has examined her and recommends the braces . . . with a $3,000 price tag! After her visit, I call the orthodontist back. "Dr. Musselman, I'm calling to try to get some sense of how necessary these braces you've recommended for my daughter really are. As far as my wife and I can tell, Laurel's bite seems pretty normal. I know that Laurel is concerned about the way her teeth look, but frankly, we hardly notice the misalignment she's so worried about. If we're really talking about spending $3,000 on something which is basically cosmetic, it just doesn't seem a good use of the money. If she really needs it, that's a different story. If her bite's going to get worse if it doesn't get fixed or if it's going to cause a serious problem later on, we would feel differently about it."

He doesn't seem to be offended by my question. "Well, I certainly understand your concern, Dr. Hilfiker, and you're right: Laurel's problem is not as bad as some. As I'm sure you know from your own medical practice, it's always difficult to predict what will become serious and what will not. Certainly, the issue may very well be only cosmetic, but there really isn't any way of telling how much worse the problem may get if we don't straighten it out . . . and it might be more difficult to do the job later. I think it would be fair to say that the primary reason for the work is cosmetic, but we wouldn't be doing it only for looks. I should add that we do have an extended payment plan. If one of your concerns is how to go about paying for the work, we could allow you to do that over several years, if that was better for you."

"Cash flow isn't really the point," I explain. "The question for us is: Is this a good use of our money? As you may know, my wife and I work with people from the inner city here who are very poor, and we feel uncomfortable using our money for something extravagant when there are so many people around us who don't even have what they need."

The conversation continues another few minutes, but although I can't be sure, I am unconvinced that Dr. Musselman really thinks the braces are medically necessary. I am almost decided against the braces.

Fifteen minutes later, however, Dr. Musselman calls back. "I've been thinking about your concerns, Dr. Hilfiker. I've heard about your clinic and the work you're doing there, and I'd like to support that. Let me offer you this: If you decide to have the work done, I would be happy to contribute $1,000 of my fee to the clinic for your work."

I am astonished, grateful for this generosity. He's caught me off guard. "Well, thank you for calling back and for your offer. That will make some difference in our thinking. I'll talk with Marja and with Laurel, and we'll get back to you."

Marja and I talk together. The need for braces still seems

to us—from the standpoint of physical health—marginal. With the exception of our car and the house we owned in Minnesota, the braces would be the largest single purchase we've ever made. On the other hand, it is hard not to see in Dr. Musselman's offer some kind of guidance for us: A third of the fee would be returned to the community and Dr. Musselman would, perhaps, feel more involved with the needs of the inner city.

Marja and I are still undecided, however. On the one hand, $3,000 is still a lot of money for us. On the other hand, if we are truthful, we *can* afford the braces. In the back of our minds is also the fear of inappropriately coercing the children onto our journey. In the end, we reach a compromise: If Laurel really wants the braces, she should be willing to share in their cost. We decide that if she will be responsible for $1,000 of the cost of the braces, we will pay the $1,000 that will be returned to the clinic as a contribution and the remaining $1,000; Laurel can use her seven-dollar-a-week allowance plus her babysitting fees to pay off her part in installments.

Laurel is understandably not excited about the idea. Like our other children, she's on her own journey, which only sometimes parallels ours. It is difficult for her to understand why we won't simply buy her the braces. Focused on getting the braces, however, she quickly agrees, and the orthodontic work begins. But almost a year later, at supper one evening, the issue comes up again, and Laurel begins to cry. She is angry.

"You don't know how weird I feel at school. Nobody else I know has to pay for their braces. All you want to pay for is 'what's necessary.' You won't even pay for my retainers."

I feel immediately defensive. Marja and I tend to be frugal—our daughters would say "Spartan"—in our spending anyway, so I don't really know how much our decision on this matter has to do with stinginess and how much stems from our real desire to be good stewards of our money. I choose defense of our stewardship as the best tack.

"We *could* pay for your braces, Laurel, but Mom and I are struggling to know the difference between what we need and what we want, and we want you to learn that, too. I know it's hard for you to live here at Christ House and go to a private school with a bunch of kids whose families are pretty rich and who get more stuff than you do. We don't want to deprive you of something really important. But the $2,000 that Dr. Musselman has charged is a lot of money, and there are lots of other places it could be used."

I'm aware that my argument isn't entirely fair. In point of fact, the $1,000 we "saved" by having Laurel pay for the braces disappeared into our regular budget, and it would be difficult to show that any of it reached the "others" who needed it. Why are we taking a stand at Laurel's braces and not at the computer I bought myself last spring "to do my writing"? There is an element of the ludicrous in my argument, and Laurel intuitively knows it. Money we save is not automatically passed on to the poor. Besides, we buy ourselves all sorts of luxuries without thinking of the poor. I'm tempted to cover my own guilty feelings over not "properly caring" for my family by making Laurel feel guilty at having so much and asking for more. I consider responding with stories of the real poverty that children her own age in the neighborhood experience. I resist the temptation.

Laurel isn't satisfied. "But if you had some other job, you'd earn more money. None of my friends understand why we live here in the middle of the city with all these poor people. Pat's parents won't let her come here after school because they're afraid of what will happen. Even Sonya thinks it's weird, and she's my best friend. She thinks it's weird that you're a doctor and we live like this, and I have to pay for my own braces. It's not just the money. I feel so weird at my school. Nobody else's dad is working for less money than he *could* get."

Laurel is angry. Part of her anger, I know, is normal adolescence: the need to define herself against us. But even though we might have made the same decision living in Minnesota, the confrontation brings back the old questions: Is our decision to come to the city really good for the children? Are we depriving them of something important, subjecting them to unfair risks? My feelings alternate between self-righteousness and guilt. I must find some way out of this.

I take a deep breath. "Laurel, let me tell you why we came here. You're right, I could earn lots more money someplace else. But I would be unhappy in those other places. Mom and I are lots happier here than we would be any other place. It's not really fair to you, but you'll have to put up with us."

As is, I suppose, usual in these arguments between parent and child, Laurel has me up against the wall. Much of what I am saying is less than completely true. Yes, Marja and I are happier here in Washington than in Minnesota; but there are many times when the stress and despair of our work get me depressed, and the kids too often take the brunt of my moodiness. Our busyness and fatigue mean that the kids often don't share in those rewarding moments when we feel more fulfilled, anyway. So I try a different approach.

"There are lots of people who live in the city who are very poor, just like the men downstairs. They don't have anything, and they deserve more. But in our country they won't get any more unless people like us help. I know you care about the people downstairs, too. The problem is, we can't have it both ways. We can't have everything we want *and* help them at the same time: We *have* to give some things up."

But this isn't quite true, either. At another time, over another issue, we *would* have it both ways. In fact, the entire project of Christ House is, in one sense, an attempt to have it both ways.

Laurel, never one to give up easily, is silent a moment. "But why my braces? Why can't I have braces?"

"Well, you can. You do! We're helping you."

"But nobody else has to pay for part of their braces!"
Perhaps it is not fair to ask a thirteen-year-old girl to understand adult decisions like ours. But Laurel listens . . .
even in the face of her own frustration.

Ever true to our principles, Marja and I slide into giving
Laurel her full allowance within a short time, "writing off"
our agreement years before she would have paid off "her
half."

Such contradictions and inconsistencies made inner-city life
hard for our kids, but they found benefits as well. As Laurel moved into high school, she would often ask me to go
over her various compositions for grammar and style. I was
surprised to discover how many times she chose to write in
one way or another about the issues raised by her life at
Christ House or by attending an expensive private school
while living so close to the poor. In a paper on Martin
Luther King, Jr., for instance, she wrote:

> Outside of school, racism is much more of an issue. A
> good example can be seen in my job at the local Burger
> King this past summer. As the only white person, besides the manager(!!!), the other workers seemed to view
> me as a snob. And I was certainly intimidated by them.
> It did not make matters any better when I was immediately put to work on the front line, as cashier, although
> this job was generally reserved for long-time employees
> who had proven themselves trustworthy. Although I was
> never told this fact, I assumed I was given this position
> because of my skin color, to give the restaurant a more
> middle-class appearance. This idea was strengthened
> when my friend [from the same upper-class school], who
> is black, began her job in "the back," although we had
> applied for the positions at the same time with the same
> credentials.

Ultimately, each of us in the family, in our own way, was
struggling with the question of justice. What was just? And

what was our responsibility as individuals when we participated in unjust structures for which we weren't personally responsible? We Americans pride ourselves on our sense of justice, but too often we do not recognize that there are different kinds of justice and that one can have a fair *process* without getting a just result. The emphasis in our country is on *procedural* justice, rather than on *distributive* or *substantive* justice—on the fair application of rules rather than the equitable distribution of goods and opportunities or the ethical ordering of society as a whole.

Take, for instance, our claims concerning "equal education." Ever since the 1954 Supreme Court decision in *Brown* v. *Topeka Board of Education*, equal opportunity in education has been national policy. No one can be barred from a public school because of race, religion, or national origin. Yet in point of fact, the education the poor receive is often vastly inferior, not because the poor are forbidden to enter top-notch suburban schools but because their families cannot afford to live in the right neighborhoods.

Consider equality in hiring: Professional jobs are, for the most part, available to all properly educated persons, regardless of economic status; but the poor are much less likely to be educated enough to qualify. Even our legal system—while ensuring fair *process*—treats the poor differently from the rich; proportionately, a far higher percentage of blacks, for instance, are sentenced to death than are whites convicted of the same kinds of crimes. Even the crimes of the poor are "less acceptable" than the crimes of the rich; shoplifting, for example, is clearly regarded as a crime, while fudging on the expense account is often considered acceptable, even though both involve stealing from businesses and evasion of taxes.

What is plain is that, while the American system may sometimes come close to procedural justice, we have neither distributive nor substantive justice in our society. Wealth, opportunity, and a good education are *not* equally available to all. Jobs open to people from an affluent background (doctor, lawyer, stockbroker, executive) pay many times more than jobs filled by those from poor backgrounds (cleaning lady, laborer, short-order cook, clerk). The courts *do* treat rich and poor differently. My relative degree of wealth is unjust: not because I earned it unfairly, not because I cheated, but because I live in a system that gives middle-class, well-educated people opportunities that the poor will never know. Since resources are finite, the collective wealth of the middle and upper classes is necessarily built on the collective deprivation of the poor.

For the most part, however, abstract issues of justice rarely move us middle-class persons to any kind of action. For one thing, against each of the conclusions above, there are deeply ingrained arguments—convincing, often, even to the poor—that rationalize and justify social arrangements as they now exist. Doctors' work, for instance, seems "more important" to us; their training is longer, therefore we feel they "deserve" a very high income. The lawlessness of the inner city seems to us to endanger our society more than the white-collar crime of government or Wall Street, even though the latter usually involves much greater sums of money, is more likely to affect every single individual (each of us has already lost over a thousand of our tax dollars to the Savings and Loan debacle while few of us will ever be robbed), and poses a greater threat to our nation's long-term economic and social stability.

Furthermore, acting justly involves concrete sacrifices, while the principle of justice remains abstract, intended to guide our treatment of people we (usually) don't know. Because I live and work in the inner city of Washington, however, the injustice done to the poor is for me no longer an abstract issue. Not only is it evident to me how the structures of our society virtually guarantee that a certain number of people will end up poor and broken, but those very people are now individuals I know—flesh and blood. The suffering here cannot be hidden. Every person in my family has been affected by it.

One night several months after our arrival in Washington, I went into nine-year-old Karin's room to say goodnight

and join her in prayers. She was crying. I asked her what
was wrong.
"I'm thinking about that homeless man we saw on the
sidewalk. You know, that one who asked us for money? He
has no place to go. Where does he get food? I can't help
crying about him. What will happen to him?"
I had no answer, so I just sat on her bed and took her
hand.
In the darkened room she looked up at me from under
the covers. "Sometimes I want to do something for them
. . . maybe go up and talk to them, maybe give them some
money. But I'm too shy."
"Some people are trying to help them," I said, and we
sat in silence for a while. Then I remembered an invitation
I'd had to visit one of the shelters. "Would you like to go
down to one of the shelters with me to see what they're
like? Maybe we can find some way you can help."
Several weeks later, when Karin and I did spend an evening at one of the women's shelters, Karin became the center of attention. One older, mentally ill woman latched onto
her, eagerly telling Karin about the shelter and asking her
questions about school and home. For Karen, mental illness
on the streets had acquired a personal face.
Once we begin to see the faces of the poor, our "sacrifices" begin to feel less arduous and more intrinsically rewarding. People regularly deny themselves certain comforts
for the sake of those they care for; it is considered quite
"normal." Indeed, it would seem strange or heartless for
parents to live in luxury while their children went without
necessities or for elderly parents to scrape by while their
grown children prospered. Giving within one's family, it is
generally believed, brings richness and fulfillment to the
giver as well as the recipient, because all are building community. At the very least, giving is a responsibility to be
taken seriously. In a similar way, when poor persons become people we know as individuals, when they are people
we care about, "sacrifice" is not the terrible thing it might
otherwise seem.

There is yet another problem in thinking of our work
with the poor or our contributions to them as sacrifices for
the sake of an abstract justice. Justice *does* demand that we
who are affluent "live more simply that others may simply
live." It is important that we be philosophically and theo-
logically clear about that demand. But on a practical, emotional level, approaching the issue of our privilege by
focusing on the *demands* of justice traps us in negativism,
in a "lose-lose" situation, and in judgmental attitudes
toward both ourselves and others. We feel guilty about our
privilege yet deprived if we give away what seems right-
fully ours.

We Americans live in an especially individualistic society. Even when people agree that they have obligations to
those less fortunate, they tend to experience those obligations as the preaching of gloomy Puritan moralism or as the
admonitions of their parents, telling them to do things they
don't want to do. By casting the demand to do something
about the overwhelming desperation and suffering of the
poor as an obligation to be obeyed, we pit ethical behavior
against self-interest and personal happiness. It's them or us!
Rare is the individual who is able (much less willing) to
yoke himself for the long haul to an abstract morality opposed to his or her day-to-day well-being and pleasure.

But within a community in which persons feel themselves responsible for one another (such as a family), it
does make sense to think of obligation as something other
than a coerced contribution; rather, it is in the obvious interest of all. Living next to the poor and working with them
on a daily basis, I've had the opportunity to understand that
we all, in some way, live together in a community and that
our obedience to the demands of justice can bring us the
possibility of a far deeper happiness, security, and sense of
integrity than can any commitment to individual wealth or
personal comfort. To the extent that I've allowed myself to
move toward a shared sense of responsibility here in the inner city, I've experienced a feeling of community that is
quite new. Marja and I have come to believe that the price

we and the children are paying to live here is amply rewarded. In the early evening, Laurel, Kai, and I are walking down Seventeenth Street to the video store almost a mile from our house. A black woman I guess to be in her early thirties approaches us. She is simply but not shabbily dressed. She looks at me deferentially. "Excuse me, sir. Could you give me eighty-five cents to catch the bus back home? I live over in Northeast, and I don't have the money to get there." I look at her directly, smile, but shake my head and continue walking. I certainly could afford to give something to her and to the others who ask me for money on the streets. But I rarely do anymore. My rationale is that I can't tell the difference between those people who will use the money for what they say they want it for and those who will use it for alcohol or drugs. (One evening near a neighboring service station I did give a dollar to a well-dressed young man who approached me with a gas can, saying he'd run out of gas . . . only to see him half an hour later drinking from a paper bag outside a McDonald's a block away.) The other option, the one Marja often chooses, is to accompany the person to the restaurant or store or bus and pay directly for what is needed, both to make it a more personal encounter and to ensure that the money is spent as claimed. But this evening I don't feel like taking the time to stand with the woman and wait for her bus, and in any case I generally feel uncomfortable checking on someone this way. I suppose I also don't like the idea of wasting my money. I try to be friendly and gentle, but I usually say no.

I pass on, but Laurel and Kai both stop. After a few steps I turn around and see them pooling their change and counting it out into the woman's hand. Laurel is talking gently to the woman. Kai's face is bright. They're obviously pleased with themselves. "It must be hard for people who don't have cars and can't afford the bus," Kai says to me matter-of-factly. "Laurie and I had *exactly* what she needed."

Even though their actions pose an implicit challenge to mine, I am pleased by my children's generosity. Clearly they have found real joy in giving something away to a person in need. From their own point of view, the eighty-five cents is well spent. I have no desire at this point to share with them my own complicated feelings and logic. Most of the lessons the children learn are complicated enough in themselves. When Kai was seven, he began playing with a boy his own age on the street and one day invited him up to our apartment. Not long after this new friend left the building, Kai noticed that his own bike was missing from the hallway. Marja and Kai asked around, and the receptionist at the front desk mentioned having seen a little boy she didn't know walking what she assumed to be his bike out the front door. Initially, Kai was upset that his bike had been stolen, but he soon found the silver lining. He'd gotten the bike second-hand, and it was now a little small for him and rattling. He'd been asking me for a replacement, and the loss of the bike gave him a stronger argument for getting a new bike . . . which he did. Kai had, it seemed to me, very little emotional reaction to having been robbed, so a few days later I asked him about it. His first response was that he could hardly believe that anyone would exchange a potential friendship for a beat-up old bike. "He must be pretty poor to do something like that." Even as an eight-year-old, Kai was recognizing that he lived in a different world from that of his neighbors. None of us ever saw the boy again.

It is in the area of family, more perhaps than anywhere else, that Marja and I confront the contradictions of our life in the inner city. When we send our children to "good schools," we often feel that we are compromising our commitment to justice. When we consider our lives at Christ House, we know we are spared the essential ingredient of inner-city poverty—helplessness. When we enroll our children in soccer leagues and ballet classes, we are aware of automatically endowing them with advantages their neighbors could not dream of.

At other times, I tell myself it is not a compromise to offer our children what *all* children deserve: a good education, a secure living environment, and a chance to develop their own gifts. That other children we know suffer from deprivation is no reason to deprive *our* children of what every child should have. There are no clean resolutions to the contradictions we live with.

More even than Marja and I do, however, our children must live between two worlds. In order to get a "good" education, they go to school with mostly suburban children of affluence. These schoolmates may worry about issues of poverty and justice; some even get involved at soup kitchens or shelters. But sometimes it can seem that in the suburbs life's problems devolve into what makeup to wear, what movie to see, how to get ahead in school, and what college to go to. Because poverty rarely intrudes, it's easy there to overlook the basic injustice of our society. But when we isolate ourselves from the poor, we do so at our own considerable risk.

The principal of Karin's private high school sent home a letter explaining why the Board of Trustees was opposing a planned halfway house for emotionally disturbed youths and young adults, to be built in close proximity to the school grounds. "We are particularly concerned," wrote the principal,

> about the 25 day-care patients who would necessarily have the opportunity to interact with our students at the facility, at the bus stop, at the Metro station, and at nearby fast food restaurants which our students frequent. At best our students would be subjected to the behavior of disturbed individuals on a regular basis. At worst, our students might be physically harmed. . . . As educators it is our responsibility to protect and to nurture our students during their most formative years.

Our children, the principal was saying, should be protected from every possible danger and unpleasantness. It is not difficult to understand the fear that these "day-care patients" might elicit in parents who have had only tangential relationships with people in poverty. One of Laurel's friends, for instance, was apparently not allowed to visit us at Christ House; while we never discussed this with either Laurel's friend or her parents, I assume that the reluctance was some combination of the fear of physical harm and the desire to protect their child from unnamed forces within the city. But there is something insidious in the attempt of the privileged to insulate their children from those with problems, from those who have not succeeded according to the standards of the society.

The difficulty is twofold. Children reared in the isolation of affluence can have little understanding of the forces that shape the lives of the poor. At the same time, these children are encouraged to believe that they have earned their place in society by their own efforts. Wordlessly reinforced is the underlying assumption that all start out on a "level playing field," but that the affluent child, by dint of hard work, discipline, and worth, creates his or her own success. When we "protect" our children from the "undesirable" elements of society, we render comparison, and thus compassion, almost impossible.

In addition, children growing up protected from others who are not like them develop a warped view not only of those others but also of themselves. If other people's chaos and confusion must be hidden "somewhere else," won't my child feel she has to hide her own chaos and confusion? If "troubled adolescents" have to be sent elsewhere, will she not fear there is no acceptable place for the troubled part of herself? By banishing those we do not understand to the ghetto, do we not banish those aspects of ourselves we don't understand into unreachable places?

Marja and I have come to believe that our children, in an enclave of affluence, would actually be exposed to greater danger than they are here, within the ghetto of poverty. Yes, there is some physical threat where we live, but any choice entails risk. Though rarely stated, the hazards of the affluent neighborhood, while certainly different, are equally real: a covetous sense of entitlement, blindness to one's privilege, numbness to the pain of the poor, and estrangement from one's own vulnerability.

Living one floor above thirty-four homeless men teaches our children that every person has worth and value despite external circumstances. Many of the men downstairs are drug addicts and alcoholics whose lives are in chaos. Yet Kai knows some of them as gentle friends. When Kai goes down to play chess with one of the men, when Karin goes to Table Fellowship with them on Thursday evening, when Laurel helps in preparing a meal, when our family joins the entire house on the roof for a picnic, my children have the opportunity to experience the possibility of community with people very different from themselves.

If the predominant and ultimately fatal illness of our culture is a numbness to the grief and pain of the poor, then our children should not be sheltered from an understanding of the real needs of those in poverty. They should have the chance to see that their education and privilege can be used for genuinely beneficial ends. Within a society where both rich and poor are ghettoized, it is simply too easy to ignore the terrifying discrepancy between the lives we live and our concepts of justice and mercy. Living with the poor, it is more difficult to remain indifferent to the suffering of one's neighbors. At least the important issues remain visible.

Chapter 7

VICTIMS OF VICTIMS

Pictures of starving children in distant lands properly evoke in us a special horror and compassion, in part because their suffering is so obvious, but also because we know that these children are not to blame for their fate. The poverty of the inner city, while no less cruel, generally elicits less compassion. It's harder to reduce to a single striking image on the TV news, and easier to dismiss as someone's fault—a single mother, an absent father, incompetent teachers, drug sellers on the corners, or an insensitive government bureaucracy. And once we can say it's someone else's fault, we can pretend it's someone else's problem, too.

Sarah Moseby sits against the wall of the exam room, sharing the chair with her four-year-old daughter, Leatrice, who is quietly sucking the joint of her bent left thumb. As I enter the cramped room, six-year-old Derwin quickly backs out of the cupboard under the corner sink with a wary eye on me. Glancing at me, Sarah bends down to swat Derwin. "Get outta there! You don't belong under the doctor's sink." Derwin jumps to one side, Sarah's swat misses, and Derwin starts pulling himself up on the exam table by grabbing at the white paper that covers it. The paper, of course, unrolls from the other end, and six feet of white paper is instantaneously curling on the floor. "Stop that," Sarah yells, and her swat doesn't miss this time.

Derwin, appearing totally unfazed by the blow, scrambles onto the table and stares up at me.

Sarah's voice is a high whine. "Dr. Hilfiker, you got to give me somethin' for him. He always bad like this. He don't pay no attention in school, and his teacher she say she gonna keep him back. She say if I don't stop him from hittin' the other kids, she don't know what to do. She say for you to give him some medicines so he won't be so hyper. The devil's got in him, I think. Why can't he be like Leatrice? She good and don't cause no problems."

Derwin's irrepressible energy is evident. He has already grabbed the end of my stethoscope and put it against his chest, tugging me down toward him. As Sarah talks, Derwin takes the stethoscope from around my neck, inserts the earpieces deftly in place, and listens first to my chest and then to his. Sarah stops in mid-sentence and grabs the stethoscope. "Put that down," she yells. "That belongs to the doctor." She turns back to me. "See, I can't do nothin' with him. He always like this. Leatrice, she be good and don't cause no problem. Gotta be somethin' wrong with him. Can't you give him some of that medicine?"

Leatrice sits passively in the chair at her mother's side, thumb in her mouth, her eyes wide, watching everything.

While I am talking with his mother, Derwin sits still on the exam table for perhaps twenty seconds and then bounces off in search of something else to do. As Sarah finishes her story, I lean down and hoist Derwin back onto the table. "Your mom seems pretty worried about what's happening in school, Derwin. I guess your teacher's pretty upset, too. What do you think about this?"

"I'm bad," he says matter-of-factly, staring with some defiance into my face. "I beat the other kids up."

"Why do you beat the other kids up?" I ask.

"Because I'm bad," he says, reaching for the stethoscope, placing its diaphragm against his chest and the earpieces in my ears. "I can beat them all up." There is a hint of pride in his otherwise emotionless voice.

"Hyperactivity" is a very specific medical condition of childhood comprising an overabundance of physical movement, the inability to maintain an attention span, and certain evidence of organic brain injury. It is a difficult-to-define, embattled diagnosis, the existence of which is not accepted by all, even in the medical community. Consequently, "hyperactivity" is also a junk category, easy to dump obstreperous children into—a simple, drug-oriented, medical "label" for what otherwise might be a messy set of social problems. By medical definition it is not a common disorder, but most of us parents at one time or another conclude that our misbehaving children are hyperactive—if only to explain their behavior to ourselves. Such is Sarah's perception. She and the first-grade teacher are unable to control Derwin's behavior: He seems unable to sit still or even stand in one place, he's constantly into things, so a diagnosis of "hyperactivity" seems obvious.

My conversation with Derwin about his problems in school and his fighting continues for a few minutes, and then I examine him, explaining everything I'm doing to him. Derwin may have a behavior problem, and he certainly has an abundance of physical energy, but it is obvious just from his ability to participate in the conversation with me and to sit quietly for his examination that he is not hyperactive. I find no neurological abnormality in my brief examination. I tell Sarah there will be no magic medicines for her child.

"Well, what can you do for him then?" she asks.

What *can* I do for him . . . or, more appropriately, for them? As is so often the case, it's not Derwin who has the problem, but his whole family. Derwin is merely the "identified patient" for a much broader set of issues, and I don't know what I can do for him or them.

Sarah has been my patient for about a year, and I am aware of the chaos in her life. Almost thirty-two years old, she is a dependent, passive person with little sense of her own powers and responsibilities. She comes repeatedly into the clinic, for instance, with *Trichomonas* vaginitis, a sexually transmitted disease that—although not serious—causes her to suffer a malodorous discharge, burning vaginal irritation, and extreme itching, while typically leaving the male partner almost free of symptoms. Treatment is straightforward: four pills need to be taken at one time by both patient and sexual partner. I have treated Sarah at least five times for *Trichomonas*, but she is apparently unable either to convince her "friend" to take the medicine or to refuse to have sex with him until he does. Her previous boyfriend, Derwin's father, abused Sarah until she finally left him. Her current friend, Leatrice's father, visits from time to time and buys Leatrice some clothes but, as Sarah's bitter complaints to me on other visits indicate, contributes little else to the family, at least financially. I believe he beats her regularly, although she refers to the abuse only obliquely and denies it when asked directly.

Sarah had lost her apartment and was up the street at the Pitts before she came to Community of Hope, where our Families in Transition (FIT) housing program for homeless families provided her temporary respite and help. The disorder of her life seems to have left her unable to follow even the simplest medical instructions without strong outside support from social workers, nurses, counselors, and others. I doubt that she is able to provide the consistent support that both Derwin and Leatrice need. I suspect that Derwin is in effect the scapegoat for a very difficult situation and becomes "the problem" within a family system that cannot cope. But I have no idea how even to begin to communicate this to Sarah.

What can I offer? I look into Sarah's pleading, distrustful eyes, and I feel overcome by her helplessness . . . and mine. "I'm not sure, Ms. Moseby. We do have a psychologist who comes in every few weeks," I suggest as a last resort, as *something* to offer. "I think it might be helpful for Dr. Wilson to see you and Derwin. He could make sure Derwin is not hyperactive, and he might be able to suggest some things you could do."

A few weeks later, Dr. Wilson interviews the Moseby

family. He agrees with my assessment and adds more. Sarah is the product of an alcoholic, abusive family and has been abandoned by each of the men she has cared for. Now, without money enough for food and rent, faced with homelessness, she can barely manage her own life, much less provide the stability and consistent discipline her two young children need. She is giving everything she possesses, every last bit of energy, to her children. There is no doubting the love and commitment she feels toward them; but it is not enough. When Derwin, sensing the chaos in the family, acts out, she resorts to the only means of discipline she knows—threats and (I'm certain) physical abuse—in an effort to control him. This punishment is imposed, however, in such an inconsistent manner that the boy has little idea what is expected of him. As a result, Derwin perceives himself at age six as "bad." He has little incentive and—given his training so far—even less ability to respond positively to Sarah's discipline.

It's not difficult for me to imagine that in ten years Derwin will be one of the young men I see slouching in the doorways of run-down buildings near Belmont Street. It's not difficult for me to imagine him, at age sixteen, as a high-school drop-out, having fathered a child or two, no prospects for legal work, a perfect setup for the drugs and drug-dealing offered at every corner in our neighborhood—if he has not long since become part of the scene, running drugs as a twelve-year-old courier. Will it then be Derwin's "fault" that he is finally as "bad" as he already thinks he is?

Child psychologist Alice Miller writes in *The Drama of the Gifted Child* that all children during their infancy need to experience the world as a friendly place and their parents as completely devoted to their welfare. What if a child is born into a world where neither parent (and too often in the neighborhoods around Community of Hope there is only one parent to begin with) has the time, energy, or emotional maturity to encourage this narcissistic phase of childhood? What if a child is born into a world where there is pressure to grow up immediately, if only to "take care of" the needy parent? That child may spend the rest of her life looking in vain for a completely devoted parent figure; and when the child becomes a parent and there is finally a person (this time a newborn) who seems to fulfill the teenage mother's previously unmet needs for love and attention, then that new baby is deprived of its own narcissistic phase as it learns to attend to the needs of the "parent." And so on, from one generation to the next.

Who is going to help Sarah, Leatrice, and Derwin become a functioning family? How will the circle be broken? While in the shelter system, Sarah will find that there are not enough social workers available even to help her fill out the paperwork for food stamps, Medicaid, or public assistance, to say nothing of people who might have the time, energy, and emotional maturity to help her approach and come to grips with her internal chaos. Even the several social workers at FIT, who can lead her through the red tape, will hardly be able to begin the intensive process of helping the Moseby family make sense of their lives or come to terms with the emotional trauma of homelessness and destitution. Once the family leaves Community of Hope, mother and children will again be at the mercy of an underfunded, desperately understaffed public system. Certainly there is no one to address the deeper problems in the life of the Mosebys.

Marr Elementary School, which Derwin has been attending since September, is crowded with children who have problems at least equal to his. Half of the students are refugees from Central America and speak Spanish as their primary language. The vast majority of the rest come from impoverished, single-parent homes like Derwin's. When our social workers visit the school, they find the teachers and staff so overwhelmed by the combat conditions that even the best of them seem able to do little more than attempt to control unruly behavior and "maintain order." Derwin has little chance of finding the long-term, sympathetic counseling and support he needs so desperately. Whom will we blame when he begins to abuse *his* children?

Mary Curran, a pastor and social worker at Community of Hope who works with the families at FIT, tells of watching children's games of make-believe on the front steps of the building. When still very young, they play at being police officers, firefighters, doctors, and teachers—all the usual roles children from "our" world choose in their games. But Mary notices that at about six years of age, things begin to change. In their games the children now begin to play addict, pusher, and narcotics agent. They play drunk; they play out fights between men and women, between parent and child. It is as if only the very young children can hold on to the dreams a truly just society might offer them; they can still see themselves as potential agents of order, rescue, healing, enlightenment—as helpers of others. The older ones have learned better. They know their future. They have begun to see what real options are available to' them. Hope has already been crushed.

And sometimes the abuse is more explicit.

Jenny was three years old when her father first brought her in to see our clinic pediatrician because of a discharge from her vagina. Routine vaginal cultures were positive for gonorrhea. Testing of other family members also found a positive gonorrhea culture in Jenny's father, who vehemently denied there was any connection. The pediatrician immediately reported the findings to Child Protection; there was an investigation, but no charges were brought and no legal determination of what had happened was entered into the record. Jenny was placed with her alcoholic mother, who was separated from Jenny's father. Within months, however, the little girl was back with him again.

Twice over the next three years different caregivers brought her in with vaginal discharges (an otherwise uncommon complaint in prepubertal children). Cultures of the vagina were always taken at these visits, but none showed evidence of infection. (These negative cultures were not strong evidence against sexual abuse; there are, unfortunately, frequent "false negatives" in which nothing shows up even when a sexually transmitted disease is present.) At each of these visits, after evaluating the entire situation, the pediatrician or nurse practitioner in charge was of the opinion that sexual abuse had most likely taken place. Each time, the pediatrician or nurse practitioner reported her suspicions to the relevant authorities. Each time she was told over the phone that without proper "proof"—culture-proven venereal disease or other physical evidence of abuse—there was little that could be done.

When Jenny is six, she is brought to the clinic with a burn on the inside of her thigh close to the groin. Her stepmother, also an alcoholic, reports that "Jenny pulled an iron down on herself." Examining the wound, Robin Wallin, a nurse practitioner with whom I work, discovers an exactly symmetrical, evenly burned triangular area about three inches across, quite consistent with a burn from the tip of an iron. It seems very unlikely that such an even burn, high up on the inside of the thigh, could have been caused by an iron falling randomly on a moving target. The wound seems much more likely to have been deliberately inflicted.

Once again we report the situation, this time to an office within the police department that deals with the physical abuse of children. The crisis worker taking the phone call is reluctant to send officers out. Without proof that the burn was intentional, she says, they can't take action. At Robin's insistence, however, a team of two workers comes to the clinic. They examine Jenny and interview both her father and her stepmother. Little more can be done, they say. Without further evidence they can't *prove* the stepmother's story inaccurate; besides, since this is the first time the situation has been reported, all they can do is make a notation in their files. Robin reminds them that we have reported the family at least three times previously for sexual abuse, and that one episode was fully documented. Their response is difficult for me to believe: Sexual abuse is reported to the sexual abuse team and is not their area. Without previous reports of *physical* abuse, they can do nothing.

Jenny still lives with her father and stepmother.

Of course, if the team from the child protection unit *had* acted—perhaps pulled the girl from the family, instigated a police investigation into the case, sent the various siblings to different foster homes for variable lengths of time, even prosecuted the parents—the results would likely only have been catastrophic in a different way. Dealing with an abusive situation requires time, energy, and resources, all of which are in short supply in the public institutions of Washington in the 1990s. The reluctance of the Child Protection workers to get involved in all but the most egregious cases is, if not justifiable, certainly understandable.

There are too many others in our neighborhood like Jenny—born to teenage single mothers; exposed to alcohol and drugs both *in utero* and at an early age; denied any opportunity for education; lacking adequate role models; abused, abandoned, and without reason for hope. How can they escape from the despair and degradation of this kind of poverty, which is so much more than economic? How can they avoid sinking into abusive and abusing relationships, alcohol, drugs, prostitution? If, as some of these children do, they maintain hope in such circumstances, it is in spite of all the forces opposing them, against all the odds, against all—one might say—reason.

The brokenness we find is often so profound it seems futile to attempt to apportion blame. Diane Baxter was only nineteen when she and her two children lost their apartment and were forced into the Pitts Hotel. Because the medical care provided by the District of Columbia at the Pitts was available only sporadically, Diane began coming down the street to the clinic with three-year-old Shawn and his younger sister, Marlene, in order to catch up on much-needed health care. Eventually the family was accepted into FIT.

Diane has some serious, probably psychosomatic health problems herself: constant, disabling headaches and a progression of symptoms from cough to chest pain to diarrhea to frequent urination for which I have been unable to find an organic cause. Such problems are frequent among homeless parents trying to cope with the unimaginable. Diane is also depressed and anxious. At Community of Hope we have tried to treat such psychosomatic problems among our patients by encouraging them to come in to the clinic frequently, sometimes to be seen by one of the medical team, sometimes just to sit in the waiting room and chat with staff or other patients. Soon Diane is coming almost every day. She tells anyone and everyone how difficult it is to take care of Shawn, especially since one-year-old Marlene alone seems to strain her caretaking resources.

From the beginning, we in the clinic notice how Shawn *is* all over the place, playing with toys, interrupting our conversations, grabbing things from his younger sister. His mother's response oscillates between two extremes. Most of the time Diane seems to pay almost no attention to him, continuing her conversation with her neighbor as if Shawn were someone else's child tearing up the place. But when she does "attend" to Shawn, Diane screams at him as if he were an adult intentionally aggravating her. She seems to have no understanding of how three-year-old children normally act. She treats every disruption as willful and premeditated.

While caring for the family, Robin has noticed that Shawn never goes voluntarily to his mother: for help, for consolation, or—as far as she can tell—for anything. One weekend Diane asks Teresa, one of the other young mothers in the FIT program, to babysit Shawn while she is away. Teresa finds it exhausting because of Shawn's high level of activity, but she becomes quite fond of Shawn, as have many of us at the clinic.

After the weekend Teresa brings him to our reception room (which at some hours of the day resembles nothing more than a day-care center) while waiting for Diane to pick him up. But when Shawn sees his mother coming, he runs and hides behind Teresa, refusing to let go of her leg, holding on, it seems, for dear life. Ultimately we have to distract Shawn with a toy so that Teresa can sneak out through the side door of the waiting room. When he notices Teresa is gone, Shawn is almost beside himself with rage.

As we talk about the issue in a staff meeting, Angela Robertson, our receptionist, mentions that Diane frequently comes into the waiting room and asks someone to hold the younger baby or to watch Shawn "just for a minute." She then disappears for several hours while the staff try to entertain the children. On a number of occasions—without asking anyone to take responsibility—she has just left both Shawn and his year-old sister in the waiting room and taken off.

There have also been reports that Diane's physical punishment of Shawn is excessive. Various members of the staff notice Diane punching Shawn with her fist, often about the head, for some real or imagined misbehavior. Her verbal threats are almost worse: "If you don't stop that, I'm going to break your arm!" When Shawn cries after being hit, Diane yells, "Why you cryin'? Nothin' happened to you," refusing even to acknowledge that she has struck him. Diane then looks at us in exasperation. "He always like this, cryin' for no reason." When we try to talk to her about her abuse, Diane refuses to respond, simply stalking out of the clinic.

Robin calls Child Protection. The worker there asks whether there are any bruises or broken bones, any physical proof that Shawn has been abused. Robin reminds her that several people in the clinic have *seen* Diane hitting Shawn, but the refrain is familiar: There is nothing Protective Services can do without "proof."

What would constitute proof—since eyewitness testimony is inadequate—is never clarified.

What is it like to grow up the child of such abuse? What is it like for Derwin to be told repeatedly by his parent that he is "bad"? What is it like for Jenny, as a three-year-old, to be forced to have intercourse with an adult? What is it like for Shawn to be struck repeatedly for what ought to be considered normal behavior? What is it like to suspect almost from the day of your birth that you are not really loved? When a person believes she is not loved, she comes quickly to believe that she is not *lovable*, and from this inescapable pain grows rage. I think of my own history. Through years of psychotherapy I have come to understand how harmful my own mother's hidden depression and the stifling of conflict in my childhood home were to my emotional health. I think of my own children: I am quite aware that my emotional aloofness, my judgmental tendency, my difficulty in expressing anger have psychologically injured them. (Will they also need psychotherapy?) My suffering, my children's suffering are real, but the emotional scars of my youth, the emotional damage I inflict upon my children pale into insignificance when I consider Jenny, or Derwin, or Shawn. If I have been made less functional by my suffering, what is the effect of theirs?

What is it like to grow up where fathers are absent from most homes and too many of the male "role models" on the streets are alcoholics, drug addicts, or pushers; where so many of the female "role models" are pregnant by the time they are fifteen? What is it like to grow up in a neighborhood where those who struggle against all odds and manage to stay off welfare and get honest employment are consigned to a lifetime of working two jobs at minimal wages just to eke out, at best, a subsistence living; where the flashy lifestyle of the drug trade is the primary example of success; where there is otherwise little hope for a future any different from the intolerable present; where the expectation of a persistent, degrading poverty pervades?

What is it like to grow up as a poor black child watching television programs and surrounded by advertisements whose basic message is that personal worth is measured by elegant homes, powerful cars, a suburban family, or sex appeal? These children, too, succumb at an early age to the myth that ours is an egalitarian system in which all start out equal and one's true merit is measured by material success. Their very poverty becomes one more irrefutable bit of evidence of their worthlessness. The dominant culture's message is starkly clear: If you were worth anything, you, too, would live in the suburbs and have all the "things" promised in the ads. These children live in conditions inhospitable to the human spirit. Is it any surprise that their usual response is to give up, blame themselves, lash out?

My thoughts turn again to my own family and to our struggles over Laurel's braces, to our prolonged decision-making process before sending Kai to the best public junior high school in the city or Karin to the same expensive private school that Chelsea Clinton would later attend. The issues my children must face and the issues these children of the ghetto must confront can hardly be compared. When I bike home from the clinic to our apartment in Christ House, I enter a whole new world.

My first responses to Jenny's sexual abuse, to Shawn's physical abuse is rage. How can parents do such things to children? I need someone to blame, someone I can hold responsible. But I have worked here too long; I have watched abused children become abusing parents, and I no longer know who the victim is.

Margine is a youngster we have known for many years. Her mother was a severe alcoholic who died when Margine was ten. During her lifetime, moreover, alcoholism kept this mother unavailable to Margine, who was moved from one relative to the next, living in constant chaos. She became sexually active by the time she was eleven . . . if it is even meaningful to talk of "sexual activity" in an eleven-year-old girl. Is not intercourse at that age almost by definition sexual abuse, and no less so because the "boyfriends" are still children of fourteen or fifteen?

In any case, all our attempts to provide her with either counseling or birth control proved futile. She even hinted from time to time that she wouldn't mind having a child so she could have someone who loved her, so she could be important in the community, so that people would pay attention to her, too. Her wish was quickly fulfilled, and soon

I was watching as fourteen-year-old Margine berated her one-year-old son for not sitting still for my ear exam, spanked him for "messin' those toys up," and neglected to bring him in for crucial medical attention. But whom could I be angry at now? Was fourteen-year-old Margine to blame? Was it her pitifully addicted mother? Or was it *her* mother, also an active alcoholic? And isn't this true for the others, too? Certainly the father who gives three-year-old Jenny gonorrhea is responsible for his behavior and society can expect him to behave differently, but do I know what *his* history is? Can I be sure that I would act differently under such circumstances (though who "I" would have been if everything—class, race, home, education—had been different from the very beginning is almost inconceivable, and that very thought of what "I" would do in such circumstances possibly meaningless)? Diane Baxter has to be held *accountable* for the way she is rearing Shawn, but can I *blame* her for treating her son in the same way she herself has probably been treated?

I think again of my own family: Marja and I were in our mid-twenties when we had our first child. We are now two parents taking care of three children. We had the privilege of deciding that I would go to work while Marja stayed home for the early years of the children's lives and gave herself full-time to child rearing. We could buy ourselves whatever material things we wanted without really pinching pennies. And *still* it was difficult to be a parent, still there were hours in the middle of the night when I thought I would go nuts if one child cried once more, *still* there was the time when I had no idea how to handle young Karin's taking money from our purse and could only seethe in frustration.

So what can I truly expect from Margine? A fourteen-year-old would have trouble being a parent under the best of circumstances . . . and Margine does not live in the best of circumstances. Life in our neighborhood thwarts all efforts to assign blame. Everyone is caught in an ugly web for which "no one" is responsible.

Is it, however, proper to speak of abusers as if they were victims? Are not all people at some point responsible for themselves? Are there not some who have endured the same background, suffered the same oppression, and yet have flowered into productive citizens? Must we excuse the poor everything because they have been at some point—or at endless points—abused?

It is true that certain individuals escape the most desperate histories to create meaningful and fruitful lives. But for the child born on Belmont Street simply to rise above the tragedy of her environment and mature into a solid, responsible citizen is an act of courage and determination at least equivalent to that of the child of affluence who graduates from high school at the top of her class and enters the most rigorous college. We do not punish the middle-class child who is merely average, yet we seem ready to consign the average child of poverty to an adulthood of misery because she cannot rise above her past. The heroes I see on Belmont Street, who—defying every predictor—manage to survive, do not obscure the reality of the terrible victimization of the rest.

John Turnell, Suggs, Bernice Wardley, Sarah and Derwin Moseby, fourteen-year-old Margine, little Jenny: Perhaps the most destructive temptation of my work is hopelessness. The poverty that confronts me daily involves a lack of money, adequate nutrition, shelter, education, medical care, and employment. It results from a society that collectively agrees it is acceptable that some people remain poor.

But if the causes of poverty were only this, I could hope. If it were simply a matter of money, food, and shelter, simply a matter of schools and clinics and jobs, I could imagine a solution. I could imagine that Community of Hope Health Services might work together with employment and housing programs like those started by others in our church and elsewhere, and that we might actually bring an end to this poverty—at least for the few people we know. A compassionate America—still the wealthiest country on earth—

might be roused to the fate of its citizens and declare a real war on those social structures that oppress and impoverish.

But in addition to that external poverty, John and Suggs and Bernice and Sarah and Derwin and Margine and little Jenny have all internalized their poverty. John can sustain his sobriety only so long; then he must destroy what he has built up and get drunk again. Suggs knows he is worthless, and—in his heart of hearts—he knows he will never get well. Derwin is quite sure he is "bad." Bernice has physical damage to her brain that does not allow of cure. Sarah and Margine, I suspect, have no sense of ever having been loved unconditionally and are unintentionally passing on to their children their own suffering. And Jenny . . . we don't know yet about Jenny. Sexual abuse in any family is a tragedy, but what happens to the child who is not only repeatedly abused but also receives virtually no education, goes hungry many days, gets her most nutritious meals at McDonald's, and lives in a large gymnasium without a shred of privacy? The damage to such lives is beyond reckoning.

In my day-to-day work as a physician, I get immensely discouraged, yet increasingly there seems to be no one readily available to blame. When I find myself angry at my patients, annoyed by their problems, irritated by some of the people I am to care for; when I find myself crossing the street or slipping out a side door to avoid them; when I find myself worn out at the end of even four hours of patient care, exhausted by the tragedy of these lives, I can no longer excuse myself by blaming them. If these are victims, *oppressed* people, those who have been "done to," on whom can I vent my frustration when their shortcomings enrage me? If my patients have been damaged so deeply, my own temporary withdrawal—however necessary to preserve my sanity and sense of self—comes to feel like an indefensible luxury.

Wherever I look I find fault—in my patients, in our institutions, in the wider society, in myself. Looking through the lens of "blame," however, is pointless. It allows little understanding and leaves no way out. To function as a phy-

sician among the poor of Washington's inner city, I have
to view my responsibilities and those of my patients in a
fuller perspective. And yet everything in our common circumstances works to obscure that view—to render the truth
of my patients' lives invisible, not only to me, but often,
I'm afraid, to themselves.

Chapter 8

INVISIBLE WORLDS

David Lawson is a mess. Thirty-seven years old, intellectually deficient, severely alcoholic with pancreatitis, peptic ulcer disease, hypertension, and a seizure disorder, Mr.
Lawson lies slumped before me in a chair. As far as I can
tell, life for him is a cycle of several weeks drinking wine,
several weeks in the hospital for treatment of his alcohol-
induced pancreatitis, then discharge from the hospital to begin again on the wine. He seems vaguely to understand that
the alcohol is not good for him, but he has little motivation
and even less ability to curtail his use of it. We have tried
to work with his "family," but the person he calls "mother"
and with whom he lives is an alcoholic aunt. The other
members of his household are an unrelated young man, apparently also severely alcoholic, and an invalid who does
not leave the house. They have not been much help to Mr.
Lawson.

Mr. Lawson moans. He looks vaguely in my direction. "I
ain't gonna lie; I had a little wine. I had a little taste." His
eyes are half-closed from the "little taste," his face grimac-
ing from abdominal pain. He looks at me again. "I'm
dyin'," he says earnestly.

He's not sure how long his belly has been hurting. In
fact, he can tell me virtually nothing of his history. He's
sure he's taking the medicines I've prescribed for him, but
when I ask him to tell me what they look like or how many

145

he takes or when he takes them, his face screws up in confusion, and he says merely, "You know, the pills you give me."

Sure that he will need to be hospitalized for yet another painful attack of pancreatitis, I examine him perfunctorily. His abdomen is exquisitely tender. He can't stand to have me touch it.

"Mr. Lawson, your pancreatitis is back. You're going to have to go to the hospital again."

His eyes widen as if surprised. "Why's that?" he asks. "Why does my stomach hurt so much?"

"It's the alcohol, Mr. Lawson. It poisons your pancreas. Your stomach hurts because the alcohol is making your pancreas sick."

His eyes widen again. "Oh," he says.

In the year that I have known him, I have sent Mr. Lawson to the hospital five or six times with the same problem, yet he is—apparently—still surprised by my explanation, still unsure what is happening to him. He tells me he "fell out" a few times over the weekend, but I can't be sure whether he means he had a full-blown seizure or just passed out from alcohol. "My mind's broke," he says. "I can't think in my head. What's wrong with my head?" I don't know whether he's been taking his medicines as prescribed, taking them intermittently, or (most likely) not taking them at all; so it's hard to know what's going on.

Mr. Lawson's medical problems would be severe enough in any situation, but they are seriously compounded by the inadequacy of the care he is offered. He does not receive Medicaid (though he is clearly disabled enough to qualify, even under a restrictive interpretation of the guidelines; his extreme intellectual disability and alcoholism have made it impossible for him to negotiate his way through the bureaucracy), so even Providence Hospital (where I have privileges) will not accept him for nonemergency care. I have to refer him to the emergency room at Howard University Hospital and hope that the ER doctors will admit him. Sometimes they do and sometimes they don't. I have yet, however, to receive a discharge summary or referral slip back after such a hospitalization. That seems almost too much to expect.

The absence of a medical summary of prior care hardly seems, on the face of it, to have much to do with the oppression of the poor, but it is one more element in the crumbling façade of third-class care. Obtaining a patient's history is by far the most important part of any medical evaluation—ninety percent of making the diagnosis and giving good care, I was taught in medical school. But Mr. Lawson's medical record at Community of Hope (like those of too many other patients) lacks major chunks of important detail because the large inner-city hospitals he finds his way into rarely manage to send us relevant records in a timely fashion. In the public clinics and emergency rooms, where cutbacks have forced an emphasis on "efficiency," the situation is even worse: Caregivers—overworked, underfinanced, wearing the blinders of their middle-class station— have even fewer resources than I do to learn a patient's history. And in emergencies Mr. Lawson must rely on ambulances for transportation, so he is taken to whichever hospital is nearest or least full, regardless of his wishes, the site of his last treatment, or the location of his doctor's practice. Winding up at a different institution each time, Mr. Lawson is once again treated by people with no knowledge of, and no access to, his medical history.

In a very important way Mr. Lawson, unable to describe his own situation with any degree of clarity and unaccompanied by any written record of the care he has already received, becomes invisible to me and his other caregivers. The particular details of his life disappear; the past that might account for the present is hopelessly blotted out, as it seldom would be for a paying, middle-class patient. To each successive doctor who cares for him, Mr. Lawson becomes just one more vagrant to move out as expeditiously as possible. After two weeks in the public hospital, he will be disgorged—pain-free, seizure-free, and detoxed—onto the streets, where the process will begin again.

Mr. Lawson's invisibility, of course, is hardly limited to the lack of medical records. He comes from a subculture I will never understand, where health is not a particular priority—one far less pressing than finding food to eat, protecting oneself from getting beaten up on the streets, or securing the next bottle of wine. Any of my usual appeals to shared values fall on deaf ears. In Mr. Lawson's surroundings, for instance, violent death is common; there is little to look forward to, and hope may have been the first victim. How can I persuade him to care about hypertension or seizure control if he can imagine no future for himself? How can I appeal to his "better self" when I have difficulty even seeing it? Mr. Lawson and I face each other over a social and cultural abyss. Because he is black, because he is poor, because he is mentally partially incapacitated, I do not "see" him in the same way I see people who are more like me.

There remains, however, a murkier cause for this invisibility, which I cannot completely articulate. I only know that when a middle-class black person or a white person of any class comes into the office, I pay more attention. I pay a *different kind* of attention. Perhaps it is simply that in these other patients I can see myself or someone closer to me. I certainly find myself identifying much more with them. While I'm not proud of it, I know also that to these others whom I can "see," I give better medical care.

It was in a small detail of my daily work that I first noticed this difference. It happens regularly in my medical practice that I simply cannot make sense of the story a patient is telling me. Perhaps it is a set of neurological symptoms that simply don't fit the way the nervous system works; perhaps it is a story of a leg swollen the day before to "three times" its normal size—now, in the office, it looks normal; perhaps it is a history of some outlandish treatment "curing" a disease. When faced with such a story, I must at some point decide whether I am going to take the patient's account at face value and continue to search for a medical, scientific, rational explanation. Or shall I push the story into some other realm: a metaphor, an exaggeration, a cultural mode of speaking, a lie, an attempt to manipulate me, or even something totally inexplicable? The question is always, "How long will I tolerate the ambiguity of the patient's complaints, how long will I persist in looking for a medical solution, before I dismiss the story as an inaccurate description of what is 'really' happening?" And there is no doubt that I will listen far longer to a bizarre story from a person of my own class and race than to the same story from a patient on Belmont Street.

There are reasons, therefore, within each of us, why I and many other doctors who treat him find it difficult to care for David Lawson. We have been too much separated. I cannot really identify with him or with his problems. Frustrated by my frustration, angered perhaps by my inability to empathize, Mr. Lawson will sometimes lash out: "I don't have to take this shit from nobody. You gonna give me somethin' for my stomach or just ask me more questions?"

And I begin to ask myself: Why am *I* putting up with this?

Even if Mr. Lawson wanted to follow my advice, he doesn't have the resources. He has neither the money nor the support from others, neither the emotional strength nor the intellectual capability that the rest of us take for granted. So the regimen I prescribe is largely ignored. We find ourselves going after him, trying to find him on the streets to give him his medicine, making incessant telephone calls to arrange for the simplest things. And when he does wander in (almost always, it seems, at the clinic's 5 P.M. closing time), drunk and in pain, I am invariably faced with the choice of resentfully caring for him after hours or guiltily turning him away to an emergency room ... that I know will not give him what he needs. Working with Mr. Lawson provides very little sense of accomplishment, and it doesn't take long for me to begrudge his demands on my energy.

To make things worse, of course, he has no money to

pay us, and—deep down—I discover some part of me refusing to understand why. I note myself feeling that it's his own fault that he's in such bad shape. It isn't that I don't know about the obvious, deep-rooted causes of poverty, or the enormous oppression facing urban black men, or even the brain damage that so severely limits this individual; but my knowledge does not seem to have much effect on my anger and resentment.

On this particular day, I stand in front of Mr. Lawson and notice not anger or resentment but a very different sentiment welling up within me: Is he worth it? Does it really matter whether this man gets better or not, whether his suffering is relieved or not? Is he worth the time and energy I am putting into him? He seems at this moment less than human, and I find myself wanting simply to send him away. Perhaps because I feel ashamed of such thoughts, I take extra care with him this day and do not leave the office until the ambulance has carried him off to yet another emergency room.

Mr. Lawson is among the walking dead of our cities. He is one of those broken people who will never enter the mainstream of American life. I could provide the best medical care, find the best housing, make available job opportunities, education, community, but Mr. Lawson's life would be little better.

People like Mr. Lawson will never be "healed" in the conventional sense, so they don't fit very well into a medical model that sees its purpose as treatment and cure or, at the very least, improving the patient's quality of life. Why am I wasting my attention on this man who will never get better? As long as I continue to deal with him, his very hopelessness becomes—in some limited sense—my own, and it's not something I want to face "for nothing."

For years on end during which Mr. Lawson made many such visits to my office, I didn't know what had brought him to his state of disability. All I saw was a mentally deficient, alcohol-addicted, seriously ill man. I assumed that most of his problem was some kind of mental retardation,

terribly complicated by his poverty and alcoholism. But trying to break through some of his invisibility and learn more
about him and his health, I finally managed (after several
years of cajoling) to get his aunt into the clinic for an interview. She told me that Mr. Lawson had been shot in the
head ten years earlier during some kind of drug transaction.
So his mental deficiency wasn't even a congenital problem, but the result of his own irresponsible behavior! A
large part of me wants to give up on Mr. Lawson. Hasn't
he brought his whole situation on himself?

It is painful to open myself up to the suffering of people
like Mr. Lawson. There is apparently so little to gain. Treating him, I have to confront my own limitations as well as
the gnawing suspicion that the poverty of many of the poor
has less to do with injustice than I had once believed. If
most of the poor are poor because of their own incapacities,
I am not so much working for justice as for charity—
providing Band-Aids for people who are incurable. Perhaps
I am even enabling them to avoid responsibility by giving
them something for free, doing more harm than good.

My work with David Lawson is not going to make *me*
feel any better about myself. Little wonder, then, that my
heart sinks when I see him for what seems like the fiftieth
time slouched down in the corner chair in the waiting room.
Little wonder that I automatically brace myself for the confusing barrage of thoughts and feelings, some embarrassing,
many that I would rather not confront, that David Lawson
and others like him dredge up in me. It's all very fine to
say abstractly that our society blames the victim and that
we shouldn't. But blaming thoughts are deeply imbedded
within me; they rise so quickly to consciousness, and the
David Lawsons of my world make such thoughts so easy to
have.

There's a litany that runs through my head in these situations: Why am I choosing to work with the dregs of society, with people who are not going to change? It doesn't
matter what I provide them. Nothing seems to get better.
Shouldn't I take my time, talents, and energy and invest

them, for instance, in children who have the potential for
change, or at least work with people who are not quite so
resistant to my efforts or, better yet, people whose problems
remind me more of my own? Even when such a flood of
questions does not surface, there's always someone—a
medical student at a talk I give; a doctor at a conference
I'm attending; my mother-in-law, wanting something better
for her daughter; a member of a congregation after I preach
a sermon—ready to ask them in my stead.

There is a belief woven intimately into the fabric of our
society that we live in a "meritocracy," a community where
people can make whatever they want of their lives, ending
up where they do largely because of their own efforts and
talents. Those of us who have "made it" often feel that we
have earned our wealth and so deserve our positions. And
since we—by dint of those special qualities of hard work,
discipline, and ambition—fashioned our own futures, anyone who does not has only himself or herself to blame.

We make exceptions, of course, for those with "disabilities." We acknowledge that society should care for the
physically handicapped or the mentally retarded, for instance, even though they do not "contribute to society" in
the usual way. But we seem to have little tolerance for
those with other, less obvious disabilities: the emotionally
ill, those scarred by early deprivation, those oppressed by
societal structures that do not allow them to develop their
full potential.

Society really does reward people according to their
merit, our often unarticulated train of thought goes; so the
poor who do not have the obvious disabilities we acknowledge must be somehow less worthy than the affluent. They
must be less intelligent, or not as willing to discipline themselves; perhaps they really *like* their condition and don't desire change enough to do something about it.

The manifestations of this belief can be seen everywhere.
On almost any news report about homelessness, for example, there is someone—portrayed as representative—who is
homeless because he or she has refused housing or hospital-

ization. In fact, the percentage of people who refuse to come to Christ House, given the opportunity, is vanishingly small. Yet observing their proportions in the news, one would think that an important cause of homelessness is the refusal of people to accept available housing. Similarly, we hear stories about "welfare queens," as if they were representative of the poor; and are reminded how many jobs go begging in the classified ads, as if most of the poor qualified for them but just didn't bother.

Even the inspirational stories about those poor people who escape their environment and "make it" within the dominant society, who become professionals, business people, or politicians, reinforce the meritocratic fantasy, conveniently ignoring the fact that the chances against "making it" from a ghetto background are overwhelming. Poor people themselves—especially those who are beginning to find their way out—often share the same distortion of the causes of poverty with the rest of us. As a culture we are deeply invested in the belief that the individual can determine his or her destiny.

In coming to Washington, I consciously rejected and fought against this notion. The poor were an oppressed people. They had had their birthright *taken* from them! They had been *forced* into their condition! But what of Mr. Lawson? Hadn't he caused his own poverty? Did he ever try to find a job? Wasn't he willing just to take whatever government handout came his way?

Margaret Mingo is a forty-five-year-old woman with diabetes and severe high blood pressure who is also morbidly obese at something over 350 pounds. She has already suffered one heart attack, but the doctors at the hospital felt that coronary artery bypass surgery would be too difficult and risky because of her obesity. I didn't see her often, but the experience was invariably the same. Twenty minutes before closing time Teresa Dyck, the nurse who works with me, would say, "David, Mrs. Mingo is here. She's run out of her pills, and her pressure is 220/130. She doesn't have an appointment, and you have two patients yet to see. What should I do?"

A diastolic blood pressure (the bottom number in the reading) greater than 120 usually constitutes a medical emergency. If the patient has any symptoms (chest pain, headache, mental disturbance, or the like), hospitalization is required. Mrs. Mingo always had at least one of these symptoms. Even without them, great care must be taken. The first several times Mrs. Mingo came in with her blood pressure so elevated, I saw her immediately, gave her emergency medication and new prescriptions, and referred her to Howard University Hospital, the nearest emergency room, for immediate evaluation. As far as I know, however, despite the many times I recommended it she *never* went to the emergency room but rather returned home and treated herself with the medications I gave her. After running out of her pills, she would wait to stop in—often for months— until she was near the clinic again.

"Mrs. Mingo," I would say, "your blood pressure is dangerously high. With your history of a heart attack, I can almost guarantee you that something very serious is going to happen to you, a stroke or a heart attack or kidney failure, unless we do something to get it under control. You could die from it at any time."

"I know," she would say. "The doctors at the hospital told me the same thing."

Sometimes I would try a different tack, thinking perhaps that I could come to understand, from *her* perspective, her inability to follow my medical instructions. "Are you having some trouble taking the medications? Is there any problem I can help you with that prevents you from getting over here? You need to take your medications every day, and I need to check you every month or two to make sure things are okay."

"Well," she would respond, answering none of my questions, "I'll come in regular from now on."

But she wouldn't. We tried phoning her when she missed appointments. We tried coaxing her to come in to the of-

fice. We had nurses visit her at home, but she soon moved
to an apartment too far away for us to continue to make the
trip. We told her we could help her find a doctor closer to
her apartment, but she said that she liked coming to our
clinic (because we were the only ones who would put up
with her erratic attendance and unscheduled arrivals?). For
a while she would send her ten-year-old son across town by
bus, then call to tell us he was coming and ask us to give
him her medications. We were then faced with the choice
of giving the boy his mother's prescriptions without really
knowing what was going on with her or leaving her with
no medication at all. And, of course, every few months she
would show up at the clinic—always, it seemed, just as we
were closing—with a dangerously elevated blood pressure.

Mrs. Mingo was not, I think, unintelligent. Why would
she refuse to make even the tiniest effort to improve her situation? She promised to come in for regular visits (and she
may well have intended to comply), but it was an empty
promise. Why was she incapable of such a simple commitment?

Mrs. Mingo's incapacity was very different from David
Lawson's. She was neither brain-damaged nor alcoholic,
but she, too, I suspected, would remain dysfunctional and in
ill health regardless of the social system in which she might
now be placed. She, too, often left me with the feeling that
she was bringing her problems on herself.

Every day I saw abused children; adolescents acting out
by getting pregnant, sliding into drug and alcohol abuse, or
simply disappearing into an urban landscape of spiraling violence; adults struggling unsuccessfully with their alcoholism or with their children. The landscape here was bleak,
and I wanted someone to blame. Perhaps there was simply
something wrong with "these people"? Dealing over and
over with David Lawson and Margaret Mingo and others
like them, I found myself confused and depressed.

Not everyone discouraged me so, of course. Rita
Branham—the young woman who, with her children, had
been squatting in the Community of Hope building when it

was purchased—was an example of an entirely different kind. Rita had been reared in a family in which all of her dozen or so siblings had severe difficulties with alcohol or drugs. When I arrived in Washington, Rita had just begun working at Community of Hope as a medical assistant, and she and her children were among my earliest patients. Little seemed to distinguish her from the other single mothers I saw as she struggled to raise her four children in the Belmont Street neighborhood. The week of my arrival she became, at age twenty-nine, a grandmother. In the office she worked diligently and efficiently. It was only later that I noticed how much people from the community trusted her, how they would share their problems with her long before they would confide in me. I soon came to rely upon her to help me bridge the gap between myself and some of those who came to me as patients.

Rita's initiative was quickly recognized by others, and we couldn't keep her as a medical assistant for long. She began to accept administrative responsibilities; she founded and directed Community of Hope's job-readiness program. In 1989, she became administrative director of Community of Hope, a position in which she remained an articulate spokesperson for the needs of the community.

In my work, it sometimes seemed that everyone I met fell into one of two categories. Some, like Rita, were poor simply because they lacked the power and money. Because they have had less impact on me, these people are clearly underrepresented in this book, even though they are a significant proportion of the patients at Community of Hope. They are willing to work hard for what they get (many hold two jobs in order to support a family); they value education for their children; they spend their meager salaries wisely; they manage to hang on to their apartments. These folks come for their appointments on time, tend to take their medicine as suggested, and return for follow-up evaluations. Sabrina Okuba, for instance, is a single mother with four children who has worked as the cook at Christ House since we began. She lives in an apartment subsidized by our housing program. In spite of a full-time job, single parenthood, and all the chaos of the inner city, she finds the energy and will to search out scholarships, enroll her children in the best private schools in the city, and see them through their struggles. All her children have attended college. Or there is Wanda Butler, who turned down the government's Aid to Families with Dependent Children for a job that pays only a little more than her AFDC check; she says she can't stand the degradation of being on welfare.

I see Patricia Chandler as a patient only during the summer. She lives on Belmont Street, but every weekday during the school year for over fifteen years she has taken the bus over an hour each way to work as a food handler in a local university's cafeteria. During the nine months of the school year, Patricia has health insurance (through a health maintenance organization), which not only pays for her doctor visits but—more important for her—also pays the price of her expensive diabetic and antihypertensive medicines. Although she has a long history of faithful employment, she is laid off every summer and her health insurance stops. Then she comes to Community of Hope. Not infrequently, we have to wait until fall to arrange the expensive medical care she needs.

It is easy for me to understand and empathize with the poverty of Rita, Margaret, Wanda, or Patricia. They have a strong work ethic, take responsibility for themselves, and seize advantage of every opportunity to make life better for themselves and (especially) for their children. Although I still cannot imagine what it is like to experience personally the severity of Washington poverty, I have seen enough of how the poor are treated to suppose that if I were in the situations of *these* poor people I would act just about as they do. I would still be "me" . . . only poor. The reasons for their poverty are clear: They have had no access to money or power.

At the other extreme are those who are poor not only because they have been excluded from the nation's affluence but also because they have, at some point, internalized their poverty in the most disastrous imaginable ways. Many of the people I see at Christ House and at Community of Hope are not only materially poor, but also can no longer imagine the possibility of anything different—if they ever could. They are perhaps drug-addicted or alcoholic, mentally deficient or emotionally ill. They are uneducated and insecure. They feel threatened, and a few are potentially violent. They can conceive of no way out of their predicament and have given up on the possibility of change.

It's no testament to my acuity that I had been working here for several years before it finally occurred to me why so many of my patients do not regularly take the medicines I prescribe, even for the most acute illnesses. Many simply do not believe that they can influence the course of their lives. Their experience has convinced them that no matter what they do, things will go from bad to worse. Their powerlessness leads to despair; they no longer believe that they can change even themselves. David Lawson and Margaret Mingo do stupid things and seem incapable of making empowering decisions. At some level I can grasp the factors that have brought them to their present situations: Mr. Lawson suffers from an impaired intellect and numerous addictions. Mrs. Mingo's health problems, her obesity, her poverty, her status as the single mother of three rambunctious boys, and her unemployability have left her with no sense of control over her life. Still, their impotence frustrates and angers me. And—if I am honest with myself—I have to admit I cannot really participate in their experience. It is too alien.

If only I could enter more deeply into their experience, I reflect, I might be able to transcend my judgmental impulse to group people into categories of those "like me" and those "too alien to identify with." But sometimes the confusion of their internal worlds is hidden behind behaviors that seem perfectly familiar: Even the fact that I don't at all understand the other person's experience is hidden from me.

Adelaid Beecher, a sixty-year-old woman referred to Community of Hope from one of the shelters, taught me well how hidden these worlds can be. The shelter supervisors refer Ms. Beecher to Ben Michael, a psychologist who works with us from time to time. If he can certify her disability, she will be entitled to Medicaid and other welfare benefits. Unfortunately, no information about the nature of her disability or her history accompanies her to the clinic, so Ben has to interview her "blind." After thirty minutes or so, looking puzzled, he comes to talk with me. "They must have made a mistake," he says. "Psychologically, she seems pretty together; perhaps she has a physical disability that isn't obvious. Could you look at her?"

I bring Ms. Beecher into the exam room and proceed to ask her about her health. No, she doesn't have any particular health problems. No, she isn't taking any medications, has never had surgery, has no allergies. She really has no complaints. I examine her thoroughly and can find nothing. At sixty, she appears in good health.

"Ms. Beecher," I say as I finish my exam, "you really seem to be doing just fine. The people at the shelter sent you over to us so that we could certify that you're disabled, but neither the psychologist nor I can find any reason that you might be unable to work. Why is it that you haven't been able to work these past years?"

"Well," she says with some intensity, "I've been waiting for my check from ABC, and they've simply refused to send it. The people at CBS have a job just waiting for me, but I'm not going to take it unless ABC sends me the check *they* owe me. I've got a job all lined up, and you can believe it pays top dollar, but I refuse to work until ABC comes through."

"I see," I say, a little taken aback. "What kind of work did you do with ABC?"

"Oh, I'm an actress, pretty well known if I do say so myself. I worked for them long and hard, but they stopped paying me. I have to get a lawyer, I guess. I'm not going back to work if they're not going to pay me."

And Ms. Beecher goes on at some length to describe her career as the star of several TV series, both famous and unfamiliar. As she begins detailing her difficulties in getting paid for her work, I excuse myself and go across the hall to talk with Ben. He seems surprised, asks Ms. Beecher back into his office, and a little while later sheepishly returns to talk with me. "She's obviously mentally ill," he says with an embarrassed smile. "But she sure knew how to cover it up when she was talking with me. You found the magic button, though. I just asked her a few more questions about her 'acting career' and she took off again." Apparently in her initial interview with Ben, Ms. Beecher—knowing she was being interviewed by a psychologist—was able to hold herself together and appear quite normal. It was only with me, the "medical doctor," that she let her guard down.

Over the next several days, the image of Ms. Beecher keeps running through my mind. Here is an older woman with a well-developed delusional system that has incapacitated her. Yet, when necessary, she is able to hide her illness from a trained and skillful psychological diagnostician. To anyone meeting her casually she appears a capable woman whose unemployment might seem the result of laziness or manipulation. But she is in fact utterly disabled by her illness. How many of the poor wander around with similar delusional systems—or mental illnesses not nearly so severe—looking for all the world like people "who just don't want to work"? And for how many others, whose incapacity is something other than mental illness, does the handicap remain nevertheless invisible, the person appearing to us simply "lazy" or unmotivated?

James Martin is a man in his mid-forties who frequently reminds me of Mrs. Mingo. Overweight, chain-smoking, hypertensive, unable to keep a job, moving with his family from one shelter to another, Mr. Martin is utterly unable to comply with the medical regimen I have recommended for him. He, too, comes in with blood pressure out of control, yet is seemingly incapable of taking his medicines, losing weight, or doing any of the other things that might improve his health. Although he never manages to make his scheduled appointments, he does drop in to the clinic more frequently than Mrs. Mingo, so we have our chance to work with him in an attempt to develop trust and encourage compliance. But *nothing* has worked. One day, completely frustrated, I refer Mr. Martin to Reginald Wilson, another psychologist who volunteers at Community of Hope, for formal testing.

As a black psychologist who worked with children in the inner city of Detroit for many years before becoming a consultant to colleges on issues of minority education, Dr. Wilson is very sensitive to the cultural biases of much psychological testing and is quick to point out the limitations of his tests. Nevertheless, Mr. Martin's overall IQ is undoubtedly in the "borderline deficient" range—a mental incapacity that he has hidden magnificently from me in all our meetings. Complicating things further, the various parts of Mr. Martin's IQ test are inconsistent with one another. His "performance IQ," for instance, is significantly higher than his "verbal IQ," indicating a limited intellectual capacity: His "street smarts" apparently guide him adequately in familiar situations, but he lacks the ability to reason his way through new ones. Mr. Martin has not appeared to me to be intellectually disabled because he does fairly well in his day-to-day life; but this is only because he functions constantly at *maximum* capacity just to get along. When it comes to taking medications on schedule or returning for appointed visits, though, he simply can't manage. His capability is overwhelmed.

It is not surprising that he has lost job after job to employers who wanted someone who would produce more. Once again, I can imagine many like him on the streets of Washington, not quite able for one reason or another to make it in our society, yet not obviously disabled either.

For reasons that I don't fully understand, I'm sympathetic to Mr. Martin and I enjoy his visits, as frustrating as the medical portion of them can be. Perhaps because he comes in more frequently, I know him more intimately; perhaps the nature of his disability is something I can understand; perhaps his earnestness and his obvious desire to follow my instructions please me; perhaps it is just personal chemistry. I find that when I can identify a specific delusion or handicap or when I grasp the nature of a limitation, my response to my patients often shifts from blame to compassion. But this fact only demonstrates my own limits. I know full well that Mr. Lawson and Mrs. Mingo have also grown up in the poverty of the inner city and that they, too, experience forces I, as an affluent person, cannot really imagine. I know that those forces shape their behavior powerfully, and I want my feelings of compassion to encompass them, too. But I don't always feel the generosity I strive for, and I slip back into the posture of blame.

Chapter 9

AVOIDANCE

At two o'clock in the morning, the telephone's ring startles me from my bed. It's Darius Miller. "Dr. Hilfiker . . . ? I'm sorry to wake you up. This is Scoop." His tone is soft, earnest, apologetic. "The nurses won't let me in. Could you let me in, so I can go back up to the second floor and sleep?"

I can't quite get my mind to function. "What do you mean they won't let you in? Where are you?"

"I'm downstairs by the door. It's raining out, and I'm cold. Can you come down and let me in? I need a place to sleep."

His voice is muffled, distant. "You're downstairs? . . . Oh, by the intercom. What are you doing there?"

But I know it's no use asking questions. In my condition, I'm not going to be able to straighten anything out over the phone. "Just a minute, Scoop, I'll come down."

I have barely set the receiver down when the phone rings again. It's from the nurses' station. I can discern Angela's lilting Nigerian accent. "Dr. Hilfiker? Darius Miller is outside, and he wants to come in. He used to be Dr. Martin's patient, but he said to call you. He said you would let him in."

"What's he doing here? Why's he calling me?"

"He just said you would let him in."

As I dress, my thoughts begin to arrange themselves. Scoop Miller is a thirty-five-year-old drug-addicted, alcoholic white man who came to Christ House six weeks ago for treatment of his bronchitis. Washington's poverty is primarily a black phenomenon; of the few homeless white people we care for, virtually all have some obvious psychiatric illness, often a psychosis, which leaves them incapable of normal independent living. But Scoop is an exception: a younger white man who did not appear to have a major mental illness. He turned out to be a delightful, almost childlike man. He remained sober and won general affection with his earnestness, his willingness to help with little chores around the place, and—to some extent—his naïveté and helplessness. He paid particular attention to my son, Kai, during Kai's frequent visits to the second floor. Scoop would tell Kai stories; they would play cards and games together; they would sometimes go for walks, often stopping to look in the window of the nearby pet store. Although I didn't know him well, I enjoyed his friendliness and his outgoing manner.

Scoop managed to remain sober during that first stay, but he showed no interest in a drug treatment program for his chemical dependency. He was sure he could handle it on his own. After Scoop recovered from his bronchitis, my partner Don Martin discharged him back to the streets. I saw him there, from time to time, and he always greeted me. Every now and then, he would even drop by our apartment just to visit Kai. Although I was rarely home, Marja would chat with him. Within the last few weeks, she had helped him find the kind of part-time job available to a street person, stuffing inserts for the Sunday *Washington Post*.

But now my sleepiness is wearing off, and I find myself irritated. Why is he bothering me? Why didn't Angela take care of this? I'm not on call! He isn't even my patient. Wondering vaguely whether I'm allowing myself to be manipulated by a drug addict or responding compassionately to a man in need, I put on my robe, go down, and open the door. A hunched shape drags itself into the vestibule, muttering almost unintelligibly, "I'm going up to the second floor."

"No, Scoop. You can't go up there. You're not a patient here anymore."

"I've been smoking PCP," he says, "and I'm afraid to go home." He looks levelly at me for the first time. His bloodshot eyes fill with tears, his pupils are dilated. He's trembling. His clothes are dirty and torn. The smell of the streets is strong in our little vestibule.

After a few seconds, he drops his eyes, turns, and reaches for the doorknob to leave.

I block his way. "Where will you go?"

"I don't know. Maybe the Laundromat across the street is open."

I just stand there. What am I supposed to do with this? I consider just letting him sleep in one of the beds on the second floor, but that would be an irresponsible decision. The institutional needs of Christ House stand in the way. I can't ask the nursing staff to handle someone who hasn't had an appropriate evaluation. I would have to do a history and a physical exam, then formally admit him. I'm not in the mood for that, nor would it be appropriate. He has no physical illness that would justify admission. If we begin admitting patients solely for the purpose of alcohol or drug detoxification, we'll quickly become a full-time detox center, unable to fulfill our primary mission. We've talked about the issue in countless staff meetings and have decided to restrict ourselves to those who are physically ill. It wouldn't be fair for me to make an exception.

But this is Scoop, Kai's friend, standing in front of me without a place to go. Marja has invested herself in him, too, and I feel some sense of responsibility. What am I to do?

It's warm for a February night, perhaps forty-five degrees, but there is a mist outside, and Scoop will need to get inside before dawn if he is to keep from getting soaked through. In our comfortable apartment, Marja, the three children, and three of Laurel's high-school friends (staying over for a rare slumber party) sleep soundly. The parents of one of Laurel's friends upstairs asleep don't even approve of their daughter coming into this part of town, much less staying at an apartment above a shelter for the homeless. How would I explain Darius Miller's sleeping on our couch to them?

I look at Scoop. His searching, reddened eyes stare back at me. Then he averts his gaze and stares at the floor. "I'm sorry I woke you up," he says quietly. "I'm embarrassed. I shouldn't have smoked the PCP. I haven't had anything to drink or taken any drugs since the middle of September, and I'm sorry I did tonight. I'm sorry I woke you up. I'll go now."

But he doesn't move. I continue to stand between him and the door. For several minutes neither of us speaks. A swirl of confused thoughts and feelings overwhelms me. (God only knows what painful thoughts are going through *his* mind!) Why can't he take care of himself? Why can't *somebody else* take care of him? Why am *I* standing here in the middle of the night? Should I welcome him in? No, isn't he responsible for himself? Isn't it *his* unwillingness to get treatment, his continued hiding from himself that have brought him to this pass? But what, then, of the abuse I know he suffered as a child? What of this terrible disease of alcoholism? Could anyone do much better in his situation? Isn't this the man "beaten by robbers at the side of the road"? But am I to be the Good Samaritan? And, if so, where's the inn to which I can take him? What refuge is there besides our own apartment? I trust Scoop sober, but can I trust him with my children and their guests after he's smoked PCP? I suddenly remember that Marcella Jordan, Scoop's social worker, and some of the others on the staff perceive Scoop as manipulative. Is he just manipulating me now? Will I only feed into his dependency by taking him in? Can I afford to take this kind of responsibility for everyone we admit to Christ House?

Standing in the doorway, I can't apportion either blame or responsibility, large or small. I can't decide what to do, or even separate my own feelings of guilt, generosity, and anger. All I know is that if I invite Scoop in, someone will have to stay awake with him the entire time, and I'm angry at the imposition.

Scoop interrupts my thoughts. "I'm sorry I woke you up, David. I'd better go."

"I guess so." I find myself hoping against all reason that he has some secret destination that will alleviate my guilt and make my acquiescence in his "decision" to leave feel less selfish. "Where will you go?"

"There's an AA meeting at seven this morning. Maybe I'll go over there." He reaches for the door handle.

I lean heavily against the door. "I'm still trying to figure out where you can go," I say. He's asking for help, and it hurts too much to let him go back into the street.

"I'd better go," he says again.

I move aside reluctantly and let him open the door. I keep looking into the eyes of a scared, hurt little boy. I follow him to the front gate. I can't send him away. But I do. And he walks into the night.

Back in our bedroom, Marja is up. I tell her briefly what has happened. Tonight was to be his first night at the *Post*, she says. Perhaps something went wrong with the job, or perhaps he couldn't resist the temptation to screw things up again. I lie down, but I know I won't be able to sleep.

After a few minutes, I turn on the light and talk to Marja again. She says she's willing to sit up with Scoop. I put my clothes back on, walk down the back stairs, and cross Columbia Road to the Laundromat; but it's closed, and Scoop is nowhere to be seen. I walk through the alley to our parking space behind Christ House, start up the car, and drive around the empty streets for fifteen minutes before giving up and returning to the apartment. It's all a futile gesture—perhaps nothing more than a pathetic attempt to salve my guilty conscience.

I argue with myself all night. Some of my arguments focus on what would be "best for him." (I can hear Marcella's voice: "You're not helping him one bit by letting him manipulate you like that.") Others focus on what would be best for me. ("You can't exhaust yourself every moment and still expect to continue for the long haul.") In the back of my mind is the recognition that the needs of the homeless in Washington are for all practical purposes infinite, and that even if I were a saint, even if I devoted every last bit of my energy to helping others, I still could not solve all the problems of this community I serve. All the arguments have a certain logical force, but the emotional reality is that I didn't take Scoop in tonight because I didn't want to be *bothered* by taking care of him all night. I'm tired, I'm stressed (a chronic condition in my case), I don't have the energy. I'm deeply moved by Darius Miller's condition, and I do not pass by on the other side without feeling pain. But I pass by, nevertheless!

Perhaps the deepest pain involved in living among the poor is the juxtaposition of my own limitations and woundedness with theirs. There are battered people all over the place! I sometimes wonder what the Good Samaritan would have done if the road to Jericho had been littered with *hundreds* of men beaten by robbers. The demands of justice, at least in this city, are endless. And it is precisely in trying to respond in some small way that I find my own damaged heart, my own limits. I can neither accept Scoop's needs joyfully nor ignore them without pain. One part of me wants to respond to every need I can, but another part is unwilling, perhaps unable. And so I remain conflicted, rarely at peace with myself.

When we discharge patients from Christ House, we offer them the option of an appointment at one of the health services for further medical help or assistance in getting drug treatment. Apparently with that offer in mind, Scoop returns to see me at the clinic several weeks after that rainy night. He is vague, but he has evidently continued using PCP and perhaps cocaine until yesterday. He is ready now, though, to go to Karrick Hall. But he will have to abstain from drugs and alcohol for at least three days to qualify for admission.

Would I admit him to Christ House so he can dry out and arrangements can be made for treatment?

I remember arguing strongly at several Christ House administrative meetings against admitting patients for detox unless they had other medical problems. Even more powerful than those rational arguments, however, is the guilt-inducing memory of Scoop walking into the night. I ignore the very rules I urged so vociferously and admit him to Christ House.

As before, Scoop adapts well to the surroundings, makes friends with most everyone, and prepares himself for the stay in the treatment program. Arranging for admission to Karrick Hall, however, takes not several days but several weeks. Finally, early one morning, Scoop gets into the van and is dropped off in front of Karrick Hall. Shortly after lunch, we receive a call from the program nurse wondering why Darius Miller hasn't shown up for admission.

Once again Scoop has disappeared into the chaos from which he came. This time, at least, I've done everything I can. *His* choosing to walk out allows me to feel less guilty for having turned him out weeks before. Even if I had taken him in, I reassure myself, the end result would have been the same.

But what would have happened to him isn't the real issue. I know what I have seen in myself, and I don't like it. My immediate response to this unflattering glimpse of my own inner depths is to throw myself once more into the fray. Overruling the limited human being I know myself to be, I decide (without consciously articulating it to myself, of course) to follow the "Mother Teresa model" of selfless giving, sacrificial service. Blaming myself for my "selfishness," I redouble my efforts. I strain to be pleasant as I see patients at our Thursday evening clinic forty-five minutes after we're scheduled to close; I struggle to finish up paperwork at Christ House in the evening rather than letting it go until the next day; I allow Helen Martin—inebriated as usual—to corner me outside Community of Hope for a curbside consultation. But I find I can't enter into the spirit of such giving with much enthusiasm. Only too soon I realize that my availability to my patients has been limited for good reason. Quickly the gap between who I am and who I would like to be proves too great to overcome, and I abandon in frustration the attempt to be Mother Teresa. "Only saints can work with the poor," I hear myself saying. In such moments, I often think about Mr. Morris and Ms. Chostek, the TB administrators from Area C Chest Clinic. Undoubtedly they, too, had once tried to offer themselves wholeheartedly to their clients—only to run into their own limitations. Had they chosen numbness and cynicism as alternatives to quitting the work altogether?

The police brought Walter McRae into the emergency room of D.C. General Hospital. They had found him unconscious on a sidewalk, one more drunk littering the streets, disturbing the view. Fifty-two years old, black, ragged, homeless, he seemed no different from countless others who find their way to the emergency room of any large city hospital. Unlike those of most disheveled men whom the police discover comatose on the streets of inner-city Washington, however, Mr. McRae's blood alcohol level was zero. The emergency room doctor saw that Mr. McRae's jaw had been wired shut, apparently at another of the city's emergency rooms.

Realizing that this was no routine alcoholic stupor, the emergency room doctors launched a vigorous evaluation and, ultimately, successful resuscitation. Although Mr. McRae's jaw had been broken, an X-ray and CT scan of his head revealed no skull injuries. Measurements of rapid pulse and low blood pressure, scant urine output, and disordered serum electrolytes led to a quick working hypothesis: After breaking his jaw several weeks earlier, Mr. McRae had gone to an emergency room, had his jaw wired shut to heal, and then had apparently been discharged back to the streets. Most likely, he had found it impossible to eat and drink enough to keep himself going, and so it was that the police found him severely dehydrated, unconscious, close to death.

Establishing the diagnosis, the doctors quickly rehydrated him with intravenous fluids and monitored his response closely: serial measurements of vital signs, venous blood for blood counts and blood chemistries, arterial blood for oxygen and carbon dioxide saturation, repeated blood draws to monitor electrolytes. Mr. McRae was admitted to the hospital, but although he seemed to be improving, his blood sodium level remained dangerously low. He was apparently even more seriously ill than he had first appeared. His condition deteriorated over the next several days until he was admitted to the intensive care unit, once again close to death.

Mr. McRae had become an "interesting case" or, as the resident doctors-in-training might term it, a "fascinoma." Teams of physicians now hovered over his chart and his withered body. Consultations were obtained from the neurology, renal, and endocrine services. All the venous and arterial blood tests were repeated, along with assays of the blood for levels of other electrolytes, various hormones, and obscure chemical by-products. CT scans and ultrasounds of the abdomen were ordered to rule out rare tumors. Examinations were repeated yet again. The consultants visited regularly. Round-the-clock nursing care with hi-tech monitoring of fluid load, heart, and lungs kept Mr. McRae going until the diagnosis could be made and appropriate treatment instituted. At last, it was clear: Mr. McRae had the Syndrome of Inappropriate Antidiuretic Hormone Secretion, an exotic hormonal disorder capable of producing life-threatening dehydration.

Intensive nursing and medical support was continued; a special ultra-low-salt diet was stipulated. The doctors scoured the city to find demeclocycline, an expensive, difficult-to-obtain medication, not routinely available at the hospital. Mr. McRae was slowly and painstakingly nursed back to health.

At the time of Mr. McRae's admission to the hospital, I was on very part-time, temporary assignment to D.C. General. I still spent most of my time at Community of Hope treating indigent patients from my neighborhood. But for a few hours a week I was serving as liaison between physicians at D.C. General and doctors at the Health Care for the Homeless Project clinics, recently established in the city's shelters. It was my job to contact hospitalized homeless patients and, if possible, ease their transition back into life on the streets. I was to review their medical charts, discuss their situations with their in-hospital doctors, arrange for follow-up, and facilitate communication between the hospital doctors and the patients' clinic doctors after discharge.

There was, of course, an element of the bizarre in such work. Mr. McRae, for example, had been hospitalized for weeks at a cost of tens of thousands of dollars, attended to by teams of nurses, doctors, and social workers, fed three carefully prepared meals a day. He was now about to be discharged to the streets, where he would sleep in a shelter, forage during the day, and wait in line in the evening in the hope simply of getting a bed for the night. How was I—who had no power over housing, food, entitlements, or any of the other myriad things Mr. McRae would need—going to "facilitate a transition" (as the job description read) back to the harshness and cruelty of life on the street? Realistically speaking, the only impact of my intervention would be that Mr. McRae's clinic doctors would have some knowledge of what had happened to him while he was in the hospital. Whether that would make life any different or any better for Mr. McRae was another question altogether.

Ignoring these disconcerting contradictions as best I could, I went to talk with the resident physicians who were caring for Mr. McRae. They explained in depth his diagnosis, prognosis, and continuing treatment. They spoke without reference to the chart; clearly, they knew their patient well. Mr. McRae was "back to his old self," they said. He would be going home in a few days ... well, not exactly *home* since he had no home, but arrangements were being made for him to stay at one of the city's shelters, and the medical team would continue to see him in the outpatient clinic.

Medicine, it seemed, could be proud of its work. Compassionate, competent care had been rendered to this homeless man without reference to his finances or social class. The medical team had not only given him the finest that American medicine had to offer, but, as far as I could tell, they had also treated him sympathetically as a suffering person worthy of attention. In my work with the very poor, I was used to stories that proceeded quite differently, and Mr. McRae's treatment gave me a rare surge of hope.

Walking into Mr. McRae's room, I discovered a long body covered to the shoulders by a single white sheet and a gaunt black face staring straight ahead. Mr. McRae's eyes were sunk so deep in their sockets that I could not even see them until—some moments after I had entered the room—he turned his head sluggishly toward me and a glazed, vacant stare slipped past me. I was shocked by the degree of his emaciation.

"Hello, Mr. McRae," I said, somewhat tentatively. "I'm Dr. Hilfiker. I work for the Health Care for the Homeless Project. I'm here to see how you're doing and if we can help you once you leave the hospital. We have health clinics in some of the shelters—maybe you've been to one—and we'd like to make sure you get good medical care once you come back."

Mr. McRae turned his head wordlessly back to its former position as if I were not there. I waited a few seconds and tried again. "Mr. McRae, I'd like to find out a little about what brought you to the hospital. Would that be okay? . . . Could I ask you about why you're here?"

There was a slight movement of the head, which I took to be assent.

"Do you know why you're in the hospital, Mr. McRae?"

After several seconds he shook his head slightly.

"Oh . . . well, do you know what was the matter with you when you came in?"

Again, a slight shake of the head.

"Well, when did you come in, then?"

"Monday." It was the first word he had spoken.

"Which Monday?" I asked after a few seconds.

"I don't know."

"I see. Well . . . uh, do you know what year it is?" Mr. McRae looked directly at me and shook his head. I moved a little closer. "Mr. McRae, do you know where you are? Do you know what this building is?"

As if he hadn't heard, he rotated his head back and continued to stare blankly forward.

What was going on? The doctors had not mentioned this side of things: Mr. McRae was not only sick but also very confused. I quickly asked a few more questions to check his mental status. Now, according to his doctors, ready to go home, he was not only disoriented as to time and place, but could not name the watch or the pen I held up to him, could not keep three different objects in his memory for even a few seconds. Mr. McRae was obviously demented.

Was it possible he was being discharged from the hospital to the street! If he could not remember the time of day or the day of the week, how would he manage to take his medicines (which in the case of this particular illness required a precise schedule)? If he had no capacity to comprehend instructions and no money with which to buy special food anyway, how would he follow the rigid diet prescribed? How could these obviously compassionate physicians send this man back to an overnight shelter in which there would be no supervision and from which he would be ejected every morning to wander the streets?

I recalled other situations in which emergency room physicians had—in my judgment—been derelict in their duty to the indigent; in which the medical problems of skid-row alcoholics had been neglected because of the bearer's social caste; in which the poor had been refused care because of their poverty. But Mr. McRae had been, medically, well treated. Why was everyone abandoning him now that his treatable condition had been "corrected"? Were there no arrangements being made to discharge Mr. McRae into a nursing home, or even a group home for the elderly? I returned to his physicians, trying to understand the situation from their point of view. No, they didn't really know what the shelters were like; none of them had ever visited one. They seemed to think of them as part of a carefully conceived network of lifeboats rather than desperate attempts to plug a ship leaking from every seam. They had no idea that the shelters lacked supervisory staff; that meals were unavailable; that ten men would be herded into a single room with cockroaches, lice, and occasional rats; that alcoholism and random violence were too often the order of the day. These physicians did not understand the cruelty of our city's "standard policy" of dumping people from emergency rooms, prisons, hospitals, and the streets into overnight shelters. In fact, the physicians had only the foggiest idea what those human dumping grounds—to which they commonly referred needy patients—were like.

But listening to Mr. McRae's doctors, I realized that the issue was deeper. When Mr. McRae had first entered the hospital, there was something that they could *do* for him. As staff at a public hospital, they could take care of this indigent man's illness without worrying about payment, and they willingly applied their energies to the task. They had the knowledge, they had the resources, and they could do some good. But that time was now over. He was "cured." There was no more "disease" to treat, and they were faced with a set of social issues for which they—as medical personnel—had hardly been prepared.

Because of a massive societal failure (for which there was no available "treatment"), there was no reasonable place to send Mr. McRae. Nursing home placement, I well knew, could take over six months, and the doctors were aware that they would soon face intense administrative pressure to discharge their patient from his expensive hospital bed. Because their honest compassion could find little scope for expression now, they had withdrawn, hardening themselves to Mr. McRae's plight and talking about discharge to a shelter as if that were a legitimate plan for a frail, demented old man who needed constant supervision. The diagnosis and treatment of Mr. McRae's real problems had little to do with the world of medicine his doctors understood. These could not be diagnosed with any medical tests or procedures, could not be treated with operations or medication, could not even be grasped with the ordinary tools of medicine. Mr. McRae's problems (now mine) required a much broader view and many more resources than his doctors (or I) could muster.

In talking with Mr. McRae's physicians, I was able to raise the issue of his dementia and convince them to keep him in the hospital until a disposition could be determined. Once I had identified the issues for them, the resident doctors needed little urging, for they were people of compassion. But like the resident physicians of whom I was so often critical, I soon lost track of Mr. McRae among the other, more acutely ill patients at D.C. General, and I don't know what ultimately happened to him. If nursing home placement was not found within an unusually short time, it is highly likely that he was discharged at the beginning of the next month, when a different set of resident doctors "cleaned house" and prepared to receive the patients who "really needed" their help.

Sooner or later, all of us engaged with the very poor do this, of course. We try to find some way of shielding ourselves from the unimaginable pain, from the inevitable failure, from the gnawing suspicion that even after all our labor things are getting worse; and our self-protective response—to become a bit colder, a bit less responsive, a bit less eager to feel the pain—becomes one more element in the oppression the poor live with every day.

Saturday evening. On call for the weekend, I've come down from my apartment to the second floor to resolve a minor problem. That's taken care of, and I sit at the nurses' station chatting with Alycia, one of the newer nurses. Two young white men whom I judge to be college students come to the front door. Alycia buzzes them in, and they walk up to the second floor. The sliding window in front of the nurses' station is closed on my side, giving me some measure of excuse for not responding to their concern, but I can't avoid hearing them as they talk with Alycia. "There's a guy out front who fell down," says one of the young men. "It looks like he's got a pretty bad cut on his head. I don't know whether he got beat up or he's just drunk." They stand expectantly at the window, waiting for one of us to get up and tend to the problem. Sensing, I suppose, that no one is very eager to respond, one adds, "The way he's dressed, he looks homeless."

I can feel Alycia glance at me as I bend over a chart trying to look busy and important. If I know one thing clearly right now, it is that I don't want to take this on. This is not our patient, I am not involved, I have other things to do, and I've been in the middle too many times before. Though I can't concentrate at all on what I'm doing, I keep my head down and my eyes on the chart.

"I guess he'll need to get over to the emergency room," Alycia says.

"He said he wouldn't go," one of the students interrupts, "but I think if someone came down and told him he needed to go, we could convince him."

Alycia again glances over at me and says hesitantly, "I guess you could call the ambulance from the phone down the hall. They could probably talk him into it."

I can now sense these college kids looking over at me, though I avoid their gaze. "We're not sure how badly he's hurt," they press. "He probably needs to be checked."

"You can use the phone down the hall. Just dial 91 to get out, then 911; the ambulance will be here soon."

They never ask me outright to come out to the street, but I'm very aware of my implicit refusal. The needs of the city are endless; a few middle-class people, no matter how well intentioned, cannot solve all the problems. I've reached my limit for this particular day. Like those whom on another day I would criticize harshly, I harden myself to the plight of a homeless man and leave him to the inconsistent mercies of the city police and ambulance system. Numbness and cynicism, I suspect, are more often the products of frustrated compassion than of evil intentions. Within most of us are wells of compassion that—given the right set of circumstances—can be tapped to liberate enormous generosity. While country folk are probably no better than the rest of us, the people in his small Minnesota town treated "Crazy Jack" with respect and attention. But when the truly broken—the chronically schizophrenic, the alcoholic, the homeless, the very poor—are herded together into ghettos; when the sheer numbers of them overwhelm us; when, by the time they reach us, they are physically unappealing, disturbed, abusive, confused, unreachable, and often visibly "ungrateful"; when the gulfs of class, race, economics, experience, and expectation separate us—then it is little wonder that we are ready to declare them beyond our caring.

If compassionate response, in addition, demands of me any redistribution of my wealth, power, or prestige, if it reveals a vision of a different society in which I am not among the "haves," the temptation to withdraw becomes overwhelming. Is it surprising that, for us who are well off, numbness so easily replaces compassion as the "natural" response to suffering?

There is another reason as well for such numbness. Many of us who have become "successful"—and this may be especially true for helping professionals—have done so at the expense of what Carl Jung calls our shadow sides. We have generally "made it" to our positions of power by repressing any sense of helplessness, suppressing feelings of impotence and rage, denying anger toward and fear of those around us, overcoming tendencies toward self-destructive behavior. Any psychologist knows, however, that those darker parts of ourselves do not go away merely because we have decided to ignore them. They continue to thrive just the other side of the thin boundary that separates the conscious from the unconscious. And—at some important level—we know those unacknowledged elements are there.

If I am honest with myself, Scoop's self-destructive tendencies are not foreign to me: I know the temptation to sabotage the plan just as I am reaching my goal. I have known within myself Bernice Wardley's refusal to deal with the reality of her dilemma, for there have been times when I refused to look at the problems confronting me, hoping they would go away. I, too, know helpless rage, though I keep it within. My self-destructiveness, my indecisiveness, my rage frighten me. They threaten both my sense of self and my chances for success. It is tempting to protect myself from my own darkness by projecting it onto those poor who suffer on the streets (and are usually a darker color than I am anyway), pretending I have nothing in common with Scoop and Bernice, making them wholly "other."

Compassion, then, brings me too close and threatens the wall separating us. I begin to fear that there is little essential difference between "them" and me. My own demons stir, and I must either avoid the suffering of the poor or wrestle with myself. If the impulse toward avoidance is so powerful for the individual, it becomes overwhelming for any group or organization: Institutions tend to sink to the level of the least compassionate response.

Within the past ten or fifteen years, our collective numbness to the tragedy of poverty has brought about a curious transition from denial to hopelessness without ever passing through that intermediate stage when personal or political indignation might lead to action. In 1984, when I first began lecturing to medical students about the abandonment of the poor, there was among them a general disbelief that such a tragedy was real. "The homeless really choose to be homeless" was a comment I frequently heard in those not-so-distant days. "If they'd just shape up, they wouldn't have to suffer so much ... It's not so bad, actually; things in the society just need a little tune-up ... The poor will always be with us; some must suffer in any society."

Talking with medical students in 1993, I no longer hear

that denial. It has been replaced by despair: Things are so bad that it is too late to do anything to help. Never grieving the loss of the American dream of justice for all, never giving ourselves the chance to feel the pain, we have gone directly from denial to hopelessness, resulting in a deeper injustice. Numbness ends up contaminating even those who do not work directly with poor people, generating a political agenda that allocates ever fewer resources to address the problems.

My living and working next to the poor gives me no opportunity to avoid the grief. I certainly know my own numbness, but I cannot wholly avoid feeling the pain.

Delores Taylor is a thirty-eight-year-old woman with severe asthma who no longer lives in the Community of Hope neighborhood. Shortly after my arrival in Washington, she moved to Anacostia in the far southeastern corner of the city, but she still travels by bus to see me intermittently at the clinic. Cynically, I sometimes tell myself that she continues coming to us only because no one else will put up with her. Her asthma is more severe and intractable than any I have ever cared for, but it is not her physical illness that gives me the most trouble. Her refusal to take medical advice even in the face of life-threatening illness drives me nuts.

I'm amazed at her willingness to drag herself in to the clinic barely able to breathe, request "a shot and a few pills," refuse my suggestion to enter the hospital, accept only the inadequate outpatient care we can administer, and take the two-hour bus ride home to suffer for weeks before returning for a shot of terbutaline (an adrenalinelike drug that can give instant relief) and a few more long-acting asthma pills. She has sometimes infuriated me with her preconceptions of which medical regimens will and will not work for her, refusing even to consider treatments that I am certain would help.

It has gradually become obvious to me—without knowing any of the specifics of her history or having, indeed, any objective evidence at all—that Delores has at some point in her life been profoundly abused and remains guarded and suspicious of anyone (within our clinic, at least) who approaches her. Her infrequent appearances in our waiting room do reflect, I suppose, the flicker of some small desire for a trusting relationship, but that desire is invariably quickly overwhelmed by fear.

In her old dress, she sits for a few minutes in the waiting room, then stands to pace the floor. If I am even minutes late, she leaves the office, not (apparently) in anger but out of an inability to tolerate her growing anxiety. She seems to be powerless to form supportive relationships and, as far as I know, has lived in lonely isolation all the years she's been coming to the clinic.

Countless times have I scheduled her for a more thorough interview and physical examination, only to have her leave without being seen, cancel at the last moment or, more often, not show up. I've also tried an alternate tack, struggling to get acquainted with her gradually on her emergency visits, asking open-ended questions, offering to do the general physical examination piecemeal. But she will have none of it. She wants her medicine (or whatever it is she's come in for), and she wants to leave.

She will not even make her refusal to cooperate explicit (which would at least ease that sense in me that I should be doing something else, something more). "I can't stay now," she'll say. "I have to get home, and you've kept me waiting too long. I'll come back tomorrow." Or, "I don't need an exam today. I'm doing fine. I just need some more of those pills." When I threaten to stop taking care of her unless she can cooperate more fully, she leaves, shunning the clinic for months, getting even less adequate care from emergency room doctors who are completely unacquainted with her deeper problems. Or she gets no care at all. After a time I resign myself to her reality and accept her back without further accusations, knowing that she—in all her disarray—is firmly in control.

Today, however, Delores has scheduled herself for an examination necessary to renew her General Public Assistance

(GPA), which provides her welfare check. A complete interview and physical examination are required. As is usually true for Delores, she's late, this time so late I assume she isn't coming at all. By the time she arrives Teresa Dyck, the clinic nurse, has committed me to see other walk-in patients in Delores's appointment slot, so it's almost noon before I take her chart in my hands and begin to think about the coming interview.

I'm irritated. One way I've discovered to protect myself from my confused and confusing life with the poor is to be definite about finishing on time. On Wednesdays, I expect to be out of here shortly after noon, and the bind in which Delores has placed me annoys me. I have a choice, of course. I can tell her to make another appointment, but this may be my only chance to get some much-needed medical information from her, and perhaps to get to know her a little better, too. I *choose* to see her, resentful nevertheless of the options she's given me. I enter the room in more emotional turmoil than I've been taught is "doctorly" or proper, hoping that, as often happens, much of my resentment will dissipate in the face-to-face encounter with my patient.

But it's not going to work out that way this time. Delores seems to believe that just because she has agreed to come to the office and sit in front of me, I will be able to fill out her medical papers without an interview or examination. She answers almost every question about her history with impatience. "Well, you can just look it up in there," she mutters, motioning to the chart in my hands (in which there is virtually no meaningful information). "I told you that all before. Or I told Dr. Goetcheus; I don't remember." When I press, she mumbles indistinctly, "I can't remember . . ." and looks down at the floor.

"You mean you don't remember if you've ever had surgery before?"

"I can't remember exactly when, no!" She sighs in exaggerated exasperation.

"Well, what kind of surgery was it? You can just tell me approximately when it was."

She sags forward again and stares at the floor. "I don't remember. I haven't had any surgery, I told you. You can just look it up in there. Why do you have to know that stuff anyway?"

"Delores, I told you before. You want me to fill out your GPA form, and that requires a full interview and physical examination to find out about your health. You have to help me if I'm going to be able to fill out your papers."

"I didn't have any surgery. I told you." A few questions later it turns out that Delores did have a uterine dilatation and curettage (D&C) some years back and a tubal ligation a few years later. But she says, "I didn't know you wanted to know about that."

I give up on the idea of getting a complete medical history.

Later I ask, "When was your last tetanus shot?"

"My what?"

"You know, your tetanus shot? They give it to you in the arm, maybe after you've had a cut or something."

"I can't remember. I never had no technical shot."

"Okay. Well, I'd recommend we give you one today. I try to remind people of it when they have their physical. If you haven't had one in ten years, you should have one to prevent tetanus."

"What's that?"

"You know, lockjaw."

"Well, I don't want no shot. I ain't taking it. I had one last year."

I give up on the tetanus shot.

And so it continues. I'm getting restless. This is a waste of time. Why am I staying late, cutting into my own personal time to go through this charade? A sharper tone enters my questions. My impatience is beginning to show.

It is time for the examination itself. It would, in Delores's case, be most appropriate for me to begin with the mental status examination, looking for elements of bizarre thinking, memory lapses, dementia, paranoia, and so forth. But Delores seems to have retreated fully into her own world. She won't answer any of my direct questions about her mental state, so I can't even tell whether some particular psychiatric illness is causing her behavior, if she is emotionally distraught, or perhaps just angry and contrary.

By this time, I'd just as soon not probe into her psychological world, anyway. The chaos there seems to me unmanageable; I would likely have no treatment for her even if I did know what was going on, and she likely would not accept it if I did have it.

I give up on the mental status examination without a struggle.

We move on through the physical examination. Her eyes now avoid mine. She obeys my requests, but stiffly and slowly, like a defiant, abused child. Teresa comes in as chaperone during the pelvic examination. Halfway through, Delores starts crying.

"I told him I didn't like this!" She spits out her words angrily to Teresa, who looks at me as if I should be able to fix things. A part of me feels like the stereotypical brutish doctor, but by now I'm so upset myself that I couldn't respond helpfully to Delores's emotional state even if I knew what to do—which I don't. Now my only goal is to go through the motions of the examination so that I can complete my task. I try to make the exam as physically gentle as possible, although I'm sure my emotions seep out the edges. Finishing, I make an effort to be polite.

But I have given up on Delores. I'm too confused and too exhausted to deal with the emotions she brings out in me, to say nothing of her deeper emotional disorder. Delores refuses even to look at me, much less answer my last questions. Whatever bit of trust may have brought her to the clinic has been shattered. I have fallen into the same trap into which every other physician she has encountered has undoubtedly fallen. The examination is over, accomplished: I have "won," she has lost. We are both estranged.

Delores Taylor does not need an asthma specialist's expertise as much as she needs a physician who will care for her, who will be with her in her pain, who will, yes, love her. It is, in fact, not so important that I do something for her as that I simply remain with her, nurturing trust between us. I came to this work precisely because I valued "being with" more than "doing for." But Delores Taylor reveals to me inescapably that frequently I don't even like the person I am to love.

Prevalent among many who choose this work is the myth that the poor are to be our teachers. Perhaps it originated in the Gospel's Beatitudes, perhaps it derives in part from Liberation Theology, but according to the myth the poor are the simple ones, the salt of the earth. Their poverty has taught them humility; their suffering has given them wisdom. We who come to "help" should learn from their elemental values, from their long-suffering in the face of intolerable odds. For the political radical or community organizer, the myth differs somewhat: "The poor" are for them the authentic source of resistance to the dominant order, the source of revolution.

These are attractive fantasies. Sometimes I find myself propagating elements of them, too.

But Delores Taylor seems far from being the "salt of the earth," and all she teaches me is how difficult caring for the poor can be, how angry I am at having to deal with her damaged self.

Those who have suffered the emotional and physical deprivation of the ghettos are not automatically "beautiful souls." It is still a shock to discover that I cannot handle the powerlessness and not even faintly edifying helplessness of the people I have come to serve. Coming face-to-face with unpleasant, ungrateful, and manipulative poor people is a misery all its own; and when I find that I cannot love my patients, or even serve them without resentment, I invariably wonder what's wrong with me. Why don't I—like Mother Teresa—see the face of Jesus in the poor? Am I missing something she sees, or have she and Dorothy Day fed me some kind of a line? Or is it possible that the poor in India are different—better perhaps—from the people I meet each day? Now I find myself not only irritated by my patients and angry at myself but also incensed at those who perpetuate these romantic myths (as I, too, have done more than once). No, I haven't found anything to celebrate in poverty—not its forced deprivation, not its denial of basic human rights, not its power to crush the human spirit.

I end up feeling that my efforts to care for my patients are too meager to be worth much. If—because of my patients' limitations—my actual medical "productivity" is minimal, if few patients end up getting better, and if our interactions are unpleasant besides, then what am I doing here? Sooner or later (usually sooner), the thought arises that I am not really suited for this work in the first place.

There are few Mother Teresas, few Dorothy Days who can give everything to the poor with a radiant joy. I am not among their company. Instead, I find myself guiltily humbled by my very unwillingness to give. In such moments, the temptation to do something with my life that "makes more sense" becomes strong.

The anger and impatience I feel toward Delores and others like her forces me to confront the unpleasant ambiguity of what I expect to get out of this work with the poor. I have not chosen to go after the enormous salaries available to physicians, and my work brings little professional satisfaction, so what kind of payment do I require? What's in it for me? Do I need Delores's gratitude to feel worthwhile? Do I need her dependence upon me to feel good about myself? Certainly her inability to adhere to any of my eminently reasonable medical suggestions means that I get slight validation of my usefulness, slight reinforcement for my "calling." Any illusions I may have of being able to really "help the poor" shatter in the face of her brokenness. So why am I here?

Some weeks after my encounters with Scoop, Christ House held a fund-raising dinner. These dinners have become a tradition at the ministries of the Church of the Saviour, joyful times when we invite staff, volunteers, and contributors

to share in the spirit of the work. We eat a good meal together and talk about our accomplishments and our plans; a
number of us—both patients and staff—attempt to describe
what Christ House has meant for us. The theme of this particular dinner was how our experience had changed our
hearts, and I knew that some of the other staff would be
talking about their encounters—undoubtedly profoundly
spiritual—with patients. But I could think only of Scoop
and me, of the exchange in all its negativity. What had happened between us? As I considered beforehand what I
would say, I realized that my struggle with Scoop served
me as an important symbol.

In the weeks immediately following my night with
Scoop, I had judged myself harshly. Despite my best intentions, I felt I hadn't opened myself, even to his most basic
needs. I hadn't been willing to give even, I sometimes accused myself overdramatically, as much as the alcoholics
on the street, who share their last drops of wine with one
another. I was hardly Mother Teresa.

But as I prepared my talk for the dinner, I began to see
things from a different angle. Scoop, I had already come to
understand, was doing the best he could with what he had,
yet nevertheless found it difficult to climb out of his history. But wasn't I also doing the best I could with what I
had? Wasn't I simply finding it difficult to climb out of my
own history?

Perhaps it was only the effect of having an audience of
people who believed in the work I was doing and in me;
perhaps it was the emotion of telling out loud the story of
my encounter with Scoop. Whatever it was, I felt tears
welling up as I talked that night. Of course I wasn't Mother
Teresa! I was just a human being harboring my own kind
of brokenness, a human being who *wanted* to be the Good
Samaritan but was as much the Levite who passed by on
the other side. As I stood speaking in the Christ House dining room, I felt almost overwhelmed by the recognition that
the pitiable person who stood before me that night in the
vestibule and the pitiable person inside me were both chil-

dren of God. If I could in my own way forgive and even love Scoop, could I not forgive myself for my own limitations? Could I not allow myself that same love? Not all of us who work with the poor are saints, but maybe we don't have to be. Perhaps sainthood isn't a prerequisite for the job.

Chapter 10

THE LIMITS OF CARE

While James Osborne, thirty-four, was sleeping in an alley doorway, an unidentified assailant—apparently at random—threw acid onto his face and upper body. His extensive and deforming third-degree burns required multiple skin grafts. His long, intensive-care hospital experience was followed by an even longer and more painful stay in the burn rehabilitation unit. Arriving at Christ House, he faces a still longer period of rehabilitation as a hospital outpatient.

Patients recovering from severe burns often wear specially designed, tight-fitting clothing: The even, constant pressure helps to decrease scarring. Mr. Osborne has a long-sleeved jacket with hood that he is to wear daily. Claiming he can't get it on, he often refuses it at Christ House, but the nurses have worked with him so that he is now—with great difficulty—able to dress himself.

Since his arrival, he's been sullen and uncommunicative. If I offer to help him put his "burn jacket" on, he yanks it away; yet on my morning rounds he complains to me repeatedly that the nurses do nothing to help him. He does not exactly *refuse* to attend the required Alcoholics Anonymous meetings or the weekly patient-staff meetings, but he is rarely in attendance, always finding some excuse for his absence. His doctors at the hospital burn unit reiterate that if Mr. Osborne doesn't use his burn jacket more faithfully, his already severe scars—large areas of pink amid the dark

189

black of his uninjured skin—will become even more disfiguring. But he persists in circumventing our efforts, all the while complaining about his disability and insisting on tending his wounds himself.

Embarrassed by his appearance, Mr. Osborne prowls Christ House, his face instinctively turned away, his body half-turned, cowed, a shadow lurking in the background. He is understandably depressed, and his depression undoubtedly contributes to his sometimes ugly behavior. He is also alcoholic. On his first night at Christ House, he returns drunk after a few unannounced hours out. I confine him to the premises for three days, informing him that if he drinks again or if he leaves the building without permission he'll be discharged. A week or so later the nurses discover him drunk again. How he managed to get the liquor into Christ House is never clear, but there is apparently an active underground among some patients and visitors. I waffle on my earlier threat, however—in part, because of some uncertainty about the degree of his intoxication; in part, because he promises with such sincerity not to drink again; in part, because I can't bear to give up on him. I tell him again that this will be his last warning.

A few days later William Mokato, the night nurse, calls me at one-thirty in the morning to examine Mr. Osborne, who is unconscious in his room, absolutely unarousable. In the wastebasket William has found two empty, pint-sized vodka bottles—apparently smuggled in, since Mr. Osborne has not, to our knowledge, left the building since I grounded him. William, of course, can recognize an alcoholic stupor, but—as is appropriate—he has called me to examine Mr. Osborne to make sure there isn't an additional cause (perhaps a head injury or drug overdose) for the unconsciousness. I dress quickly, remembering my midnight drives to the small hospital emergency room in Minnesota, thinking how convenient it sometimes is to have my patients living downstairs. I check Mr. Osborne briefly. He is simply drunk.

I don't deliberate very long. I feel honestly sorry for him

as I write the discharge orders, for I don't know how he is
going to care for his burns on the street. He can sleep it off
overnight, but he'll have to leave in the morning. I go back
to bed.

Around noon the next day Peggy Cuthburtson, one of the
volunteer nurses, who's been living and working with us
for a year, calls me at the clinic during lunch hour. "James
won't leave, David. He's pleading with me to stay. I told
him you had ordered his discharge, but he seems so sad, so
sincere. I don't know what to do with him. I can't just
throw him out. Would you come over and see him?"

On my return, Mr. Osborne seems a changed man, and
I'm not surprised Peggy wants me to reassess my decision.
Instead of the sullen, morose noncooperation I expected, he
offers me directness and honesty. He looks me straight in
the eye as I walk into the room and says in apparent can-
dor, "Look, Doc, I'm sorry about what happened last night,
okay? I should never have done it. I won't let it happen
again. I promise." His face is bright and expectant. He has
done his part, it seems to say, confessing and apologizing;
now I should do mine.

I feel torn. Everything seemed so obvious last night. I
understand very well that, for the sake of the other patients,
the staff, and the institution itself, we must establish and
enforce unambiguous rules governing the kinds of behavior
we will tolerate at Christ House. The patients need to know
the limits of our tolerance in regard, for example, to violence, so that they can feel physically safe with the other
men, and they need a structure within which to struggle
toward their own sobriety. The staff needs to know clearly
what the rules are, so they can interpret them consistently
to the men. I need to establish boundaries to preserve my
own sanity.

To those of us who work here, the rules about alcohol
use certainly seem important for the mission of Christ
House. Mr. Osborne knows those rules and has already
been given one chance and an additional "last warning."
But what if he really has experienced some kind of conver-

sion? Might he not be sincere? Isn't it possible that my leniency this time would help generate the trust so important in finding a way out of his alcoholism and other troubles? These are the times when I fervently wish that my position lacked all authority.

"I'm sorry, Mr. Osborne, I really am, but that's what you told me Monday morning. We simply can't allow you to stay here if you're going to drink. Too many others are trying to stay dry, and your drinking makes it a lot more difficult for them. I warned you last time. I'm afraid you'll have to leave."

The expression of a reprimanded child spreads over his face. His eyes plead with me, actually brimming with tears. "Where am I supposed to go, Doc? How am I supposed to take care of these burns? You know I can't get this burn jacket on without help. Just give me one more chance. Try and forgive me, and I'll be all right. You gotta let me stay here. I can't go out on the street looking like this!"

Now what? Mr. Osborne's pleading pierces me. He even uses the language of Christ House, which I know—and he has learned—so well. Should there be no "forgiveness" for this man? I want to see Christ House as an institution of hope, and I am used to taking long shots, often choosing to trust on the least shred of hope. Has he got another chance coming? Or is this just one more con?

Peggy is standing next to me, and I feel a responsibility to her and the rest of the staff. They're the ones who will have to handle Mr. Osborne's behavior on a day-to-day basis after he's secured his readmission and I'm out of sight. I feel a responsibility to the other patients. I know, for example, how difficult it is for Mr. Osborne's roommate to stay on the wagon. If we don't make it very clear, by enforcing the rules, that alcohol is not allowed, those who are committed to changing themselves will not receive the support they need from us. I know that the patients use our every inconsistency to justify their own problems.

"I'm sorry, Mr. Osborne, you'll have to leave. I'll be happy to see you at my office over on Fourteenth and

Belmont. I'll try to help you from there, but we can't take
care of you here. Your things are in your bag. You'll have
to go."
   I walk out of the room. As I leave, his voice trails after
me, pleading. "Please, Dr. Hilfiker, you've got to give me
one more chance. I thought this was a Christian place . . .
I can't go out on the streets with my face like this."
   Peggy and I walk in silence to the nurses' station. I try
to read her expression. "What do you think?" I ask weakly.
"We have to let him go, I guess. Do you have any sense of
it?"
   Peggy shrugs uncomfortably. It will be my decision. He
will leave.
   But if my verdict is unequivocal, my feelings are not.
Where will James Osborne go? Will his wounds become infected without proper care? Are our strict rules about alcohol a moralistic rigidity, an unfair, middle-class attempt to
control the "unruliness" of the poor? Am I being fair to Diane, the nurse who has been working most intensively with
him and believes they are beginning to establish a trusting
relationship? I am casting an ill, damaged, homeless man
back onto the streets. Is this why I came to Washington?
   From one point of view, of course, my guilty feelings
show just how far out of touch one can get, working in this
environment. Mr. Osborne has had his warnings. He is not
a child, and he is responsible for his own behavior. At
whatever level these decisions are reached within the addicted person, he's made his choice; and, in any case, regardless of how responsible Mr. Osborne is for his actions,
his drinking has serious practical consequences for the other
people in Christ House. From a logical standpoint, the decision is clear.
   But logic is not the only consideration, and often not—
within my work context—the strongest. Whatever brought
him to the streets in the first place, Mr. Osborne now lives
a breath away from tragedy. As I, in some small way, share
his life, the immensity of that potential tragedy comes per-
ilously close.

To what extent is James Osborne responsible for what he does? Does it make a difference that he has been damaged by forces far beyond his control? The traditional teaching of Alcoholics Anonymous assumes that addicted persons must—if they are to change—face the consequences of their own behavior. But the potential impact on Mr. Osborne of such "tough love" is many orders of magnitude greater than even the loss of family or job that a middle-class person might risk. Is it hopelessly naïve to imagine that one more experience of trust and forgiveness might enable James Osborne to free himself of his history?

Because he lives so near the edge, I, too, must peer into that same abyss: Any of my decisions can be a matter of life and death for him. How can I not err on the side of extreme caution, allowing him to stay unless the situation is crystal clear . . . which it will never be?

At issue is the paradox of any limited institution working against problems that are essentially limitless. In a just society, there would be other options besides violating institutional structures or condemning sick alcoholics to the streets. Because of the societal abandonment of the poor, however, a choice between such meager options is frequently demanded. The objective reality is that the wider society is responsible for turning James out into the street; the subjective reality is that I am. And the saddest thing is that his bed will be occupied so quickly that I won't even have much time to feel guilty.

If my own attitudes and feelings vacillate so extremely when I consider a patient's alternatives, the issues become almost impossible to resolve when other staff members, struggling with the same questions, mix in. My first patient when I return to the clinic after lunch is Jacinto Mendez, drunk as usual. I've seen him repeatedly at the clinic in the past eighteen months and hospitalized him more than once for the consequences of acute and chronic alcoholism. Jacinto, forty-two, is a Cuban refugee who came to the United States with the Mariel Boat Lift. Somehow Jacinto made his way to Washington and joined its growing Hispanic community, becoming a familiar and—in his often brightly colored clothes—sometimes comical street figure in our neighborhood.

Jacinto belongs to a cadre of Cuban alcoholics who once claimed as their "home" the wide entranceway to the abandoned building that was to become Christ House. Christ House was *his* home long before it was mine. In any case, Jacinto is technically not homeless. Several years ago Martha Butler, one of the clinic social workers, was able— because of his chronic heart failure—to obtain for him a disability determination under the Supplemental Security Program (SSI) of the Social Security Act. Martha then became Jacinto's "representative payee," which means that she receives his SSI check and makes sure he gets at least the basic necessities, using part of the money to pay rent on a room that she also found for him. But Jacinto seems always to be on the street somewhere, usually hanging around Christ House. He's perpetually intoxicated, coming into the clinic sometimes to get his "daily" dose of seizure medication (he seldom manages to take it without supervision), sometimes to have his head sewn up after a fight or a fall, or occasionally for treatment of a serious illness.

A year ago Jacinto was gravely ill from alcoholic cardiomyopathy: His chronic alcohol use had caused irreversible damage to the muscle of the heart, leading to heart failure. He barely survived and spent weeks in the hospital. Given the precariousness of his heart condition, especially in light of his continued alcohol abuse, he has done fairly well. Today, he has come in complaining of a painful boil on his back, which—from a strictly medical point of view—is a relatively straightforward condition, needing only a simple incision, drainage, and twice-daily antibiotics, which we can administer from the clinic when we give him his seizure medication.

But all is not so simple. Jacinto is so intoxicated it's likely he doesn't grasp what I'm suggesting and, even if he did, would probably not manage to get to the clinic on schedule for his medications. I consult with Martha, and after some discussion we decide she will call the city detox unit to take him for a few days until he sobers up (during this time *they* would be responsible for administering his antibiotics). Afterward he might enter a longer-term alcohol treatment program or, at the very least, be better able to manage his medications.

It turns out, however, that Jacinto has worn out his welcome at detox. He has been down there so often in the last few months that the intake workers refuse to consider him again. Although highly placed city health officials later assure me that no one is ever turned away from the detoxification center, it is—by our personal observation and experience—common practice for the detox staff to refuse admission to some of the street people who go there regularly.

Martha returns to my office and closes the door behind her. Her face is drawn, almost rigid; her voice is shaking. "They won't take him down at detox, David. I've done everything I know how to do. You tell me no hospital will admit him without a serious acute illness. Detox won't take him, he won't go into the long-term alcohol treatment program at St. E.'s, the receptionists here are getting tired of his stumbling in every day and bothering everyone else in the waiting room." I wait for the question I know is coming. "Can't you admit him to Christ House for a few days?" Her question is almost defiant.

Here we go again, I think to myself. All I need is Martha on my case! For the second time in as many hours, painfully conflicting feelings arise around a coming refusal, this time complicated by Martha's emotional involvement. I find myself becoming cool, almost withdrawn.

"Martha, you know Jacinto isn't really homeless. He *has* a place where he can go. There are lots of men out there who could use some time at Christ House, but the staff has made the decision to limit admission to people who really are homeless. Besides, I don't think Jacinto's infection is that serious. If he'll come in here for his medications every day, I think he'll get better quickly. I'll see him here. If he doesn't come in, we can go out and get him."

It's not difficult to read her anger, her frustration with Jacinto, and her despair at the unwillingness of Christ House to do anything for him. In our staff meetings at the clinic, we've talked about Christ House and twenty-four-hour care for the homeless so often that many of the staff have begun to see Christ House as the solution for every hopeless case they encounter. I know Martha looks at Christ House as a place where Jacinto should be able to dry out, get gentle care, good meals, and rest, and have his skin infection treated by competent nurses.

"Nobody else will take him, David. Now you're telling me you won't admit him, either. What's the place for, anyway? Jacinto needs to dry out, or he'll never get better."

"Martha, it's not my fault that Jacinto is drinking himself to death, and it's not your fault either. You're not responsible for making things okay for Jacinto. Part of working here is learning to accept that there are tragedies we can't do much about. We have to do the best we can and then let go." I recognize that concern for Martha is only one of my motives. I'm also maneuvering.

"Well, what's he supposed to do, then?" Martha's face is flushed now. She's not about to let her welfare be my excuse for avoiding this situation.

"Martha, admitting Jacinto to Christ House isn't going to solve anything. He really needs detox and long-term alcohol rehabilitation, but there's nothing like that available, especially for someone who doesn't speak English. He wouldn't accept it anyway. Christ House isn't a detox center. You know what Jacinto is like when he's detoxing. It isn't fair to ask the nurses to deal with that twenty-four hours a day. They're burning out as it is. If I admit Jacinto for detox, I'll have to take in every other drunk in the city, and soon we'll be a full-time detox center."

"*They're* burning out! Well, what about me, David? What about Jacinto? You aren't the only ones who can burn out!"

I'm frustrated with having to defend myself. "I don't know, Martha. I can't solve all the world's problems. We've done what we can. You've already gone the second mile with him, maybe the third. We can't do any more. He can't come into Christ House."

Martha glares at me, turns abruptly, and walks off without another word.

I'm left feeling awful. At some level, I understand Martha's frustration and her unwillingness to accept my reasoning. At some level, of course, she understands my position, too: the nightmare of triage in a city where there are insufficient resources. But her anger, her implicit accusation that I'm insensitive to Jacinto's condition, trigger feelings I'm not eager to deal with for the second time in so many hours.

There is no good solution to Jacinto's problem, and that is neither Martha's fault nor mine. But with this man at this moment, I am ready to acknowledge that I can't do everything, that I will have to let some things go. Martha, on the other hand, has invested much energy in Jacinto. She knows that, outside of Christ House, there is nothing else to be done, and she feels responsible for what happens to him. At another time, our roles may be exactly reversed. But for the time being I have become an agent of the system, one more door slamming shut in Martha's face.

Jacinto Mendez and James Osborne appear incapable of taking care of themselves. Even a few such patients would be hard to handle, but here in Washington there are thousands, enough to fill scores of Christ Houses and still leave the local health care system overwhelmed. Little wonder that in this world of neverending demands, we who would offer care find ourselves so threatened by chaos. In a limitless situation, it becomes necessary to set limits, to decide what we will and won't do, what we will and won't allow. The need to establish "appropriate" boundaries is perhaps our most painful task.

It is common for helping professionals to feel responsible for meeting their clients' every need. And because our clients' needs are so enormous, it can seem particularly selfish to hold back, to keep anything for ourselves. On the other hand, since much of current pop psychology discounts the very possibility of healthy self-sacrifice, it can be difficult indeed to sort out the differences between a "healthy" giving, born of our deepest desires to love, and an "unhealthy" giving, springing from unfulfilled psychological needs—for approval, for achievement, to appear "more saintly" than we really are. But if we don't make that distinction, if we attempt to follow unrealistic models of selflessness, we all too often (and all too suddenly) find our feelings of concern turning into hostility. Alcoholics and addicts can be masters of manipulation. Many know intuitively how to take advantage of our desire to help, how to make their needs become our own, how to exacerbate our alternating feelings of guilt and resentment, blame and anger. If we force ourselves to respond to all the needs we encounter in a day—to say nothing of a week, or a year—we can quickly end up feeling embittered, angry, resentful. Then, on the rebound, guilt over such less than saintly attitudes can make us feel like so many Scrooges on Christmas Eve. And these internal conflicts are greatly intensified when our own strong emotions clash with those of another, equally well intentioned colleague.

Every year interns come from across the country to live and work at Christ House. The volunteers are mostly young, well educated, and white; frequently they are recent college graduates working for a year through church-related voluntary service organizations. Sometimes they live at Christ House itself, sometimes in an organized community with other volunteers elsewhere in the city. Most often they come to gain another kind of experience and perspective before continuing their educations or professional lives. In my work with them, I often saw journeys that reminded me of my own, though greatly compressed in time.

These volunteers encountered the same lives I did, confronted the same obstacles. We met together every Thursday morning to talk about what was happening to us and how we were responding. The process was predictable, unmistakable. During the initial few months (while they were meeting the thirty-four men who, at any time, are living at Christ House; while they were experiencing poverty for the first time), there was much optimism. The work was difficult but challenging. When the volunteers became frustrated, they could usually project their anger and confusion onto the society that had oppressed the men or onto the system at Christ House, which was somehow not responsive enough. When, during these early months, I would suggest that some of the despair and depression the volunteers were experiencing might come directly from the nature of the homeless themselves, and revealed a part of my own negative feelings toward the men, I could feel certain volunteers' impatience. Few articulated it, but it was not difficult to sense their disappointment in me. How could I blame the poor for their plight, "write them off" so willingly, and limit myself and my availability so severely?

A few months later, with a much fuller awareness of the men at Christ House and their problems, the volunteers sometimes lost track of the injustice that had created this state in the first place. Now, when the volunteers were frustrated, they were often angry with the men. I, meanwhile, became no longer a cynical old man but a Pollyanna who couldn't fathom the depth of the betrayal they were experiencing. During these months we often had our most productive discussions. A few months more, however, and the volunteers were beginning to question *themselves*—their motivation and their competence. It was a very recognizable pattern, this shifting of blame from society to the poor to the self. The final, and perhaps most difficult, passage of their journey brought them to an understanding of the limitations of us all.

The anguish of the volunteers may have been the most obvious sign, but in truth all of us at Christ House were embarked on the same journey, albeit at varying speeds. Our journeys were parallel but not synchronous, and so we would find ourselves irreconcilably at odds, with deep emotional investments in the positions we took.

It is my weekly meeting with the volunteers. Our talk this morning has been especially distressing. Lois Harper cannot even articulate her pain, her sense of betrayal. She is a registered nurse who has already volunteered eighteen months of her life at Christ House without pay. In return for full-time work, she receives only a tiny room on the third floor—large enough for a single bed, a small desk, and an easy chair—and meals taken with the men downstairs. She is a gentle, contemplative young woman who feels a calling to the religious life and who has come to work with us out of those strong convictions. Lois is loved and deeply respected by many of the men for whom she cares.

Because she usually works evenings, Lois is also the nurse who most often has to confront men who have gone out drinking or drugging or have stayed out beyond the 9 P.M. curfew. She has drawn her share of blood samples for alcohol testing, collected her share of urine samples for drug testing. For some men she has been the point of primary contact with the discipline of the system.

Last weekend George Mifflin was admitted. George had stayed with us several times previously but had never been able to stop drinking. Twenty-four hours after his admission this time, he returned drunk on Lois's shift, and she confronted him. George left angrily, discharging himself before we could act.

The pain of George's leaving, of her "failure" to reach him was bad enough. But when Laura Shapiro, the head nurse, learned the next day about the circumstances of George's departure, she angrily accused Lois of lacking understanding and compassion and of overstepping her authority. Laura believes strongly that everyone who comes in deserves every chance to recover, to reform himself. She almost always sides with the needs of the individual patient and would not discharge anyone for drinking unless his behavior was particularly obnoxious. Laura feels it is her own

mission—and, by extension, that of Christ House—to provide grace and forgiveness to those who have been broken
by the system. In reality, her outburst probably had little to
do with Lois (who wasn't even responsible for George's
self-discharge) and was more likely an expression of her
frustration with an institution that seems to her more severe
than it ought to be.

For Lois, the primary result of the confrontation is confusion over what constitutes the appropriate setting of limits. Probably because of their own mixed feelings about the
matter, Laura and Lois never discuss the incident again, but
Lois's sense that she should have done more, been more
compassionate, could have prevented George Mifflin's exit
to the street, remains with her. Laura's angry reproach and
accusation of hardheartedness catch Lois at her most vulnerable.

Both Laura and Lois are compassionate. But as they
struggle with the difficulties of their work, it's easy for
them to end up venting their frustrations on each other. It
is not that Laura was right or wrong in her response to
Lois. It is rather that when staff members have to make decisions together, or to deal with the results of one another's
decisions, the underlying pain and insecurity of working
with too many people who seldom "get better" is sharply
heightened.

"I have to get out of here," snaps Melanie Morris later
in the same meeting. "I can't stand working here when nobody tells me what's going on. I thought we had a rule
about alcohol. I thought we agreed in team meeting that if
Jack Billings came in drunk, we were to discharge him. So
he came in drunk last weekend while I was charge-nurse. I
confronted him and told him he'd have to leave in the
morning. Then Laura comes in and tells him he gets another chance. It makes me look like an ass. I tell him he's
going to be discharged, and then he gets to stay. Two days
later, he comes in drunk again. Now it's the doctor who
comes in and says the patient is 'too vulnerable' to survive

on the streets. How do they expect me to work down there if I don't know what's going on?

"And then last week, there was Bill Wolfe! I was just getting to know him. We had a good relationship, and I think he was starting to make some new decisions about his life. It felt good to me. That's why I first volunteered to come here, to develop some meaningful relationships with people like him. So on Thursday night he has alcohol on his breath, and he's discharged before I even come in the next morning. Everybody knew how I felt about him, but nobody thinks to ask my opinion. He never got a second chance . . . while others like Billings have come in drunk or high a dozen times and still get to stick around! What's going on?

"It seems to me," she continues, without waiting for an answer, "that all that stuff about rules is just a smoke screen. If you're the social worker, or the head nurse, or the doctor, *you* get to decide whether any particular man is going to be allowed to drink or use or come in late. If you're a peon on the floor, you have to live with it. It's no wonder the men can't figure out what we're talking about; there really aren't any rules, just personal responses of certain people that determine things."

What Melanie is running up against is an institution struggling to deal with an impossible situation. One option for a program like Christ House—an option frequently chosen by governmental agencies that do work similar to ours—is to have explicit rules and adhere to them absolutely. At many of the halfway houses for addicts in Washington, if you use once, you're out! Christ House, too, has a formal policy prohibiting the use of alcohol or drugs. Unfortunately, relapses are part of the disease of addiction, and a rigid, legalistic policy is incompatible with the humanitarian impulses that brought us to this work in the first place. Regardless of our rules, we find it difficult to discharge a man who has been waiting for six months to get into a special rehabilitation program and "slips" the day before he is to enter it. We find it impossible to discharge to the streets a frail, demented, and ill man who happened to wander outside and accept a drink from someone on the street.

Like many other voluntary institutions, we try to take "individual needs" into account. We want to be free to bend the rules for the sake of the needs of the person before us. The end result, however, is that at times we seem to have *no* effective institutional policies at all; in the case of an infraction, staff members are left to decide the appropriate response with only their feelings to guide them. Our desire to individualize policy becomes as confusing for the patients as it is for the staff.

The same institutional difficulties in setting limits arise in our relationships with local hospitals. Christ House was founded as a *temporary* medical shelter for homeless men who needed short-term medical care unavailable on the street. It's a highly specific mission. The hospitals we work with also have clear missions, but they often find themselves caring for patients whose acute medical crises have been resolved but who then become, like Mr. McRae, "disposition problems." Uninsured, unable to pay, in need of permanent nursing home placement, these patients may be severely demented or chronically ill. They may have some form of mental illness from which they will never recover enough to live independently. Yet though most of the nursing homes in the District of Columbia are required to treat the indigent, the wait for a bed is long: It can take up to six months to thread a patient through the needed certifications and bureaucracy onto the appropriate waiting list and finally into a home—very expensive months for the hospital forced to provide interim care.

Hospital social workers, who quickly catch on to the difficulties institutions like ours have in setting limits, begin subtly threatening to discharge this patient or that patient to the streets if he is not accepted into our program. These are not, of course, empty threats; hospitals discharge some very disoriented patients to the streets, and many of them die of cold, neglect, disease, or abuse. So those responsible for deciding who is to be admitted to Christ House often find themselves caught amid the very specific mission of Christ House, their own sympathies, and the chronic needs of their community.

But there is no simple solution. In opening itself to the chaos of the streets, Christ House, too, becomes vulnerable to chaos. It is not surprising that we frequently do not know how to respond.

Chapter 11

POVERTY MEDICINE

The absence of clear guidelines is virtually the hallmark of medical practice among the poor. "Poverty medicine" sometimes seems related to the rest of American medicine but more often it plunges me headlong into a world for which my medical school training never prepared me. There are, of course, varieties of poverty medicine: Doctoring in Appalachia will look different from doctoring in Washington, will require one set of skills in a Harlem walk-in clinic and another in a Florida migrant worker camp; nevertheless, these varieties have more in common with each other than any of them do with mainstream American medicine.

It is not the diseases that are different. Though heart disease and cancer kill a disproportionate number of poor people, the illnesses are the same in the suburbs as in the inner city. Because they frequently lie concealed behind well-constructed façades, addictions to cocaine or alcohol are less noticeable in upper- and middle-class neighborhoods, but substance abuse with all its consequences is a part of any physician's practice. Though the stresses of suburban and inner-city life may be very different, the stress-related illnesses—headaches, stomachaches, back pain—are the same on Belmont Street and in rural Minnesota. The strictly medical, scientific training a doctor needs to practice among the very poor is essentially the same as preparation for any other primary-care practice.

It's not the science that is different.

Kathy Bartlow is a severely alcoholic, forty-year-old white woman in our neighborhood. Sober, she is one of my favorite patients, actively attending AA, trying to help her neighbors, earnestly working toward her own recovery. Drunk—as she is this particular afternoon—she is a nightmare.

Kathy has a seizure disorder, but I have never been able to determine whether all of her "spells" are genuine seizures. The regularity with which she starts twitching and shaking whenever I begin to refuse some drunken demand of hers seems more than coincidental. Today she wants to go to Sibley Hospital to "dry out." A year ago, when she came to the clinic with pancreatitis and impending delirium tremens, we finagled her admission into Sibley, a wealthy, private hospital in far-northwest Washington that had recently agreed to accept a small number of nonpaying patients from our clinic. Kathy loved it. Now, a year later, she has decided for the umpteenth time to quit drinking and—although she has no acute physical illness at this point—wants to be readmitted to Sibley for detoxification. Since Sibley is not a detox center but a hospital that, as an act of charity, allows me to admit the occasional indigent patient, I feel I can't risk alienating the hospital staff by admitting Kathy (who is loud and demanding when drunk) just for detox.

"I don't think that'll work out, Kathy. The hospital is just for when people are sick. What you need right now is detox. Let me call down to detox and see if they have a bed. Maybe Lois could take you down there."

She sits disheveled in the corner, her short, tight skirt muddy and pushed up high on her thighs. Spittle hangs from the corner of her mouth. She straightens up and teeters on the edge of her chair, trying to look me in the eye but seeming to lose focus. "I ain't going to that hole. I

wanna go o'er ta Shibley!" She slurs her words in what
seems like a parody of drunkenness.
I notice that the side of her face is beginning to twist and
distort. "Well, I don't think that'll be possible, Kathy. But
we have to get you help somewhere."
She suddenly screams, "You gotta help me, David!" Still
sitting in the chair, she lunges forward, grabs my hand, and
hangs on hard. "You gotta help me." She stares into my
eyes and then loses focus. Suddenly she lets out a grunt,
halfway between a moan and a curse. Her face stiffens in
a hideous grimace. She flops back in her chair and begins
sliding down to the floor. (Is it only my cynical imagina-
tion, or she is gently lowering herself with her arms?)
Reaching the floor, she seems to position herself carefully
with her head between the chair and the wall and then begins shaking irregularly, spit frothing on her lips in what is
either a seizure or a remarkable imitation of one.
I've been through this before.
I call Lois to stand guard while Angie phones for an ambulance. Fifteen minutes later the rescue squad appears. By
this time Kathy is up once again and hanging on to Lois.
As I come into the room, she lurches toward me, clumsily
hooking an arm around my neck. "You gotta send me to
Sibley, David. I can't go on like this." On seeing the rescue
squad, she squeezes my neck in a violent bear hug. "I love
you, David. I love you. Don't let them take me. Don't let
them take me." Suddenly she flops back in the chair, and
her seizure, or whatever it is, begins again.
Members of the rescue squad, dressed in the rubber suits
of the fire department (in Washington, firefighters are the
first to answer *all* emergency calls), have been watching
through the door. "She did that last time," says a tall white
man with a mustache. "She can really put on a good one.
She started scratchin' my eyes out when she got to the ambulance. You call the police. I'm calling the ambulance off.
We ain't takin' her again."
Kathy is still shaking on the floor. "She needs to go to
detox," I say.

"Well, then, you call the police. That's their department."
Within a minute they're gone, and I ask Angie to call the
police.

Angie buzzes me right back. "They said if she's having
a seizure call the ambulance. They won't take her if she's
having a seizure."

Kathy soon passes out in the exam room, while I do my
best to see other patients. Harlaney Pearson, the medical assistant working with me this afternoon, watches over Kathy.
Fifteen minutes later Kathy decides she'll come back "a little later" and stumbles out of the office.

One of the first things a doctor of poverty medicine gives
up is the power the physician wields within the American
medical system. Kathy Bartlow, my patient, has come into
the office asking—at some level—for healing. But I have
the power to accomplish next to nothing. I can spend hours
with Kathy and yet be unable to provide what I would have
considered in Minnesota the most basic medical care. The
way the police and ambulance systems work in the inner
city is not responsive to the needs of the poor—or their
doctors—so I sometimes don't even have the power to get
my patient transported to the hospital. In Kathy's particular
case, I *do* have the authority to admit her to Sibley, but
must use that authority sparingly for fear of alienating the
institution or even having that privilege taken away. What
can I offer Kathy Bartlow?

What *did* I offer Kathy Bartlow? What did she receive in
this encounter that accomplished nothing? My undivided attention. My respect for her and for her heartrending struggle. My willingness to be there, to listen, and to offer what
little I had: to call the ambulance, to protect her from immediate harm (at least for the few minutes she was with
us), to care whether or not she got better. I find frequently
that those are about the only things I can give my patients.

I spend an hour with Maggie Walker, a thirty-three-year-
old heroin addict who desperately wants out. Her family
has fallen apart, she is facing jail, and she is being threat-

ened with having her children taken away from her. She is
willing to "do anything to get clean," but there is no inpatient drug treatment available in Washington for addicts
who have no insurance or other means of payment. All
that's available is a public methadone clinic where Maggie
would be seen for a few minutes daily as an outpatient to
receive a narcotic substitute for the heroin she is already
taking. As far as the rest of her life is concerned, she will
remain in her drug-infested neighborhood; she will receive
only minimal psychological help or group support to help
her break her habit; she will get no practical assistance with
the insurmountable problems that confront all poor people—lack of housing, security, work, cash. Even the methadone clinic, the sole program accessible to her, has a
waiting list five weeks long. Although I'm her doctor, I
can't open the door she so desperately wants to walk
through. She and I know full well—though neither of us articulates it—that in five weeks, when her appointment at
the methadone clinic comes up, the moment will have
passed, and she will be in no shape to take advantage of it.
The time is now; but there is nothing I can do. I can only
maintain hope (against our shared hopelessness), offer my
presence, and try to introduce some modicum of concern
into an environment in which it's so often absent.

For all my supposed authority as a physician, I have only
a little more power than my patients to improve the conditions under which they live. I may be able to diagnose
Vaneida Thomas's hypertension, but I can't offer her an
apartment, get her kids out of trouble with the police, get
her a job, protect her from an enraged boyfriend, or provide
her the tools for fashioning a new and healthier life. I can
tell Donald Marshall why and how he should change his
diet and take his insulin, but I can do nothing about the inadequate education that prevents him from understanding
the diet, or about the economic obstacles that, in any case,
make it impossible for him to buy the appropriate foods. I
am powerless to affect his despair, his certainty that nothing

a doctor could suggest would fundamentally alter his life or his options.

Lois and Teresa and I work for months with the Roberts family as they search for housing with the "assistance" of the city's various programs for the homeless. Mr. Roberts is severely, often psychotically, depressed, in real need of hospitalization; Mrs. Roberts has a borderline-low IQ and life-threatening diabetes that—though she is only in her thirties—has wreaked havoc throughout her body. The family, homeless for months, has passed through the shelter system several times. Medical care has been virtually impossible. They come to the clinic infrequently, take their medicine sporadically, under stresses that make control of diabetes, to say nothing of depression, a fantasy.

Mr. Roberts finally finds housing for the family, but six weeks later he reports that the landlord refuses to fix a multitude of defects that render the apartment almost uninhabitable. It is winter; windows are out, the plumbing doesn't work, and the back door can't be locked. The apartment has been broken into once already in their brief tenancy. When the Roberts family was at the city shelter, their fifteen-year-old daughter was sexually assaulted, so now Mr. Roberts stays awake all night to guard the unlockable back door. Mr. Roberts tells us that the landlord wants the family out, and it seems likely he is (illegally) refusing to maintain the apartment as a means of pressuring them to leave. No one within the city system responds to Mr. Roberts's complaints or pleas for help, and within two months the family finds itself in the shelter system again, having "voluntarily" (according to the social worker's report) left their apartment. During this time Mr. Roberts has given his wife insulin only from time to time, if at all, and she has been hospitalized at least three times for dangerously high blood sugar. I am as helpless as they are to find them housing or redress even a few of the injustices and humiliations they suffer.

On Belmont Street, health is not so much a question of disease. The strictly medical factors are rarely the most crucial to healing. While a patient's lifestyle and environment are important elements to be considered in *any* medical evaluation, traditional medicine nevertheless finds its power by breaking problems down into their constituent parts, isolating individual issues and dealing with them as discrete clinical entities. But the complex, interrelated web of troubles that confront the poor make it impossible for me to treat the medical portion of their lives in isolation. I cannot address James Martin's hypertension without worrying about his economic status (how is he going to fill his prescription?), his educational level (does he understand the need to take medicines—especially given their side effects—that will not, in the short run, seem to do anything for him?), or his family situation (how does the incarceration of his oldest son or the pregnancy of his daughter affect the hypertension?).

Within traditional medicine, the physician is the central player because he holds the keys to wellness. The doctor who chooses poverty medicine, however, not only finds his own power circumscribed by the same forces that dominate the lives of his patients but also quickly discovers that he is not the most important player on the team. At any given time, it may be the nurse, the social worker, the nurses' aide, the counselor, or the receptionist who offers what is most needed.

Defined by usual medical expectations, the "success rate" in our practice is abysmal, and inevitably so. As a physician, I know how to treat high blood pressure. It's not difficult, but it requires regular office visits, a certain familiarity with basic medical language, patients' compliance with treatment recommendations, money for medication, and the ability of patient and physician to work problems out collegially. When patient after patient returns to the clinic with blood pressure wildly out of control, it's sometimes hard to remember that my patients' medical failures are not always and necessarily my own professional failures.

I am speaking to a group of university medical students and faculty about the living and health conditions of my patients. I can sense that the stories are touching the hearts of many of the students and young doctors. During the question-and-answer period at the end of the session, a distinguished professor of pediatric surgery, garbed in a long white coat, rises and says earnestly, "I can only applaud your commitment to the poor, Dr. Hilfiker, but don't you think it's a waste of your professional education? Why should a person go through four years of medical school and at least three years of postgraduate hospital training to take care of problems that are so obviously social and societal in nature? It seems to me that your job might better be done by a social worker or nurse practitioner, while you used your talents more effectively elsewhere."

The surgeon, I suspect, is trying to persuade his students and residents not to "waste" their own educations by choosing work as "useless" as what I do, but he articulates the doubts any doctor whose patients are poor people will experience: Am I throwing away my education and training, possibly letting my competence erode? What if—after years of this kind of practice—I get to the point where I am unqualified to be a "real doctor"?

In clearer moments we who practice poverty medicine are aware that the surgeon's questions and our self-doubts are only part of the story. It takes all the medical judgment we possess to discern when to let go and when to press a homeless patient. It takes every bit of our medical authority to get such patients into the health care system. It takes as much medical knowledge as we can muster to diagnose across cultural barriers. But—since our work is so different from a doctor's standard routine—it is easy, from the medical point of view, to mistake it for no work at all.

At a practical level, the usual professional support systems—continuing education, journals, conferences, societies, and academies—have not yet been developed to meet the needs of a physician who has decided to work with the poor. There are professional associations for gastroendoscopists and medical journals for ophthalmologists specializing

solely in diseases of the retina, but there is no Academy of
Poverty Doctors, no *Journal of Poverty Medicine.* There is
no curriculum for poverty medicine: no one teaches "The
Art of Medical Decision Making with Limited Funds" or
"Medical Compromise within Cultural Strictures." Medical
practice in a community of poor people often seems a solitary specialty without research, common cause, or shared
experience. I and my few partners are isolated professionally, with no way even to assess our own record.

In a culture that measures success and competence in
dollars, it's easy—when the stresses of practice become
overwhelming—to feel that a relatively low salary is further
proof of professional lack of worth. The same goes for
prestige: As a physician for the poor, I know there will be
no "professional advancement." The bottom rung of the
ladder is the same as the top rung: working as a clinic doctor, seeing patients day-to-day.

Looked at from one angle, the limitations this environment imposes require an almost indecent compromise of
professional standards. From another perspective, however,
we who practice in poor communities are in the process of
creating new "medical" approaches to dilemmas the profession has too long ignored or mishandled. Most of my patients have already, after all, fared badly in the traditional
medical system and are often disinclined to submit to standard procedures like interviews and examinations, not to
speak of expensive tests for vague or minor complaints . . .
or even for serious ones. A new art of caring is needed for
the poor.

Mr. Tanner, an elderly gentleman with anemia and intermittent traces of blood in his stool over the past six months,
arrives at the clinic today for a visit . . . but only because
Teresa called him and insisted that he come in for
follow-up. "No," he says of the colonoscopy I've been rec-
ommending every visit for the last six months, "I think I'll
wait a little on that bowel test." I explain for at least the
third time the danger of bowel cancer, doing whatever I
know how to impress on him that blood in the stool is a

dangerous sign and that such a cancer would threaten his
life. But he looks down at the floor, hems and haws, mumbles something under his breath. If he would even let me
off the hook by refusing my request outright, it might be
professionally easier; that is, he could help me create a
more recognizably middle-class medical exchange, in
which individual decision and individual responsibility—his
and mine—are clearly delineated.

"I'll need to think about it," he says and smiles, almost
mischievously. "Maybe I could check the tests again in a
month or two. Maybe it'll be gone."

"Even if the stool samples are okay the next time," I argue, "it's important to have the colonoscopy because just a
single stool sample with blood in it can be a sign of danger."

He looks up triumphantly, "Well, I sure don't want to get
that bowel test if we don't find no blood there. I'll let you
know."

Six months from now we will have the same conversation.

Joanne Davis is a young, homeless mother. She is diabetic, taking an insulin injection once a day, but her blood
sugar is not well controlled. I have suggested a somewhat
complicated but commonly used schedule for insulin administration (a mixture of short- and long-acting insulin,
split into morning and evening doses). Because Joanne, fortunately, has Medicaid, we are able to get her a home glucose monitor (a small machine about the size of a handheld
calculator, which determines her blood sugar level from a
strip of special paper impregnated with a single drop of her
blood); but she is apparently unable to use it regularly. Although she gives no excuses—in fact, she won't even admit
that she hasn't used it regularly—I can imagine that living
with two small children in shelter conditions of minimal
sanitation, having to pack her belongings up daily to lug
around the city, and lacking any sense of what the near future (or even the day) holds for her family makes my medically "sensible" program a hopeless task. To keep the

insulin refrigerated, the supplies intact, and the monitor from being stolen, to say nothing of maintaining a diabetic diet or finding motivation to draw blood two or three (ideally four) times a day, might be beyond anyone's powers in Joanne's circumstances. In addition, she has a visceral dislike for giving herself shots and so "forgets" to take her evening dose on a regular basis. After struggling with her for several months, I finally agree to revert to less effective single daily doses of insulin and periodic blood sugar checks at clinic visits (which she will often miss anyway). So her blood sugar levels remain far from ideal, and she is at high risk for serious complications, or even death, at a relatively early age.

The first few times I met with Joanne, early in my career in Washington, I was frustrated by her situation. I redoubled my efforts to get her onto a "proper" regimen. After she again and again failed to reach the goal I thought we had set together, I began to retreat, labeling her a "tough case." When the next diabetic patient came in, I energetically encouraged him to use the more difficult but more effective treatment. But having tried unsuccessfully to convince patient after patient to accept that regimen, my enthusiasm for insisting on the "proper" treatment wanes. I notice that when a new diabetic patient begins resisting my suggestions, I settle more rapidly for what, by usual medical standards, would be considered less than best.

I am torn. I know what "good medicine" is: I practiced it for seven years in northeastern Minnesota. From the perspectives of the academicians in medical school, the specialists downtown, or even other primary-care doctors only a few miles from Belmont Street, I am not meeting the standards of good medicine. Since those are perspectives I share, it is painful to look at myself and my work through their eyes.

The realities of the ghetto, however, demand a new set of standards—not "lower," but simply more appropriate to the environment of poverty. It is not reasonable to expect

Joanne Davis to keep bottles of insulin refrigerated while moving from shelter to shelter; to hold on to a supply of insulin syringes when clean needles sell for three dollars each on the street; to eat three well-balanced meals a day with snacks in between; to draw blood for monitoring four times a day. Such expectations only demonstrated how far out of touch I was with her reality. My job is, in part, to help her find the appropriate compromises between the conditions of her life and the dictates of "good medicine."

Oncologists on the cancer wards or geriatricians working with people in the last years of their lives have also had to develop standards of medicine particular to their work, but these standards have already been accepted by the rest of the medical community. The things I commonly do to care for my patients, however, are still too often seen as "bad medicine," difficult to justify to other doctors, difficult to defend in a court of law, difficult to rationalize (even to myself, a product of very traditional training), especially when the inevitable—if rare—bad outcome and threat of malpractice litigation occurs. It is of little solace that indigent patients are less likely to sue than are middle-class patients.° My fear of practicing "bad medicine" persists.

I can look at my choices and realize that my willingness to meet my patients "where they are" makes medical care accessible to people who might otherwise get nothing. The ability to accept such compromise and work with it is a necessary qualification for a good doctor of poverty medicine. But deep within me, there is always the gnawing fear that I am not so different from other incompetent doctors— those who prescribe tranquilizers for every complaint, those who are not sufficiently discriminating and treat even serious organic disease as "psychosomatic," those who have not kept up with the important developments in medicine.

° Almost all physicians believe that poor people bring malpractice suits against their doctors *more often than* affluent people do, despite the lack of data supporting this belief and several studies and reports that suggest poor people sue less often.

Too often I am aware only of my failures and find it difficult to take pride in my "specialty."

This fear is, of course, a form of suffering, suffering any
doctor has to accept as an inevitable aspect of practicing
medicine with the poor. Such feelings of vocational frustration, of professional helplessness—my inability to do what
I want to or know I should do—in some small way help me
grasp the vast frustration, anger, and lack of self-esteem of
my patients, whose deprivation makes my anxieties seem
trivial, who suffer horrible abuses, who are not likely ever
to achieve the dreams they have for themselves or their
children.

I don't see Marjawn Dixon very often. She doesn't seem to
be able to make it to the clinic for regular appointments, so
I am surprised this Thursday evening to see her sitting in
our corner exam room. Marjawn is forty-four years old, and
I know very little about her. She misses every appointment
I schedule for a more thorough interview and physical examination, and she usually says very little in the office. I
take her chart from the rack beside the exam room door and
read what Teresa has written. Ms. Dixon's blood pressure is
220/140, disturbingly high.

I walk into the little exam room. Ms. Dixon is a thin,
dark, black woman in a plain, threadbare dress. As I appear,
she seems to shrink into the chair, as if she hoped I
wouldn't notice her. She never looks at me, but stares
blankly at a spot on the floor.

I recognize the familiar posture right away, and I'm uncomfortable. How many of my patients stare at the floor
when they talk to me! I feel like an absolute monarch before a subject. Is this one more legacy of slavery? Or is it
another manifestation of class structure in our officially
classless society? I don't like this position of dominance. I
want her to treat me as an equal. Her eyes, riveted on the
floor, upset me.

But I restrain myself. "I'm glad you came by, Ms.

Dixon. I've been worried about you. How've you been doing?"

"Fine."

"The nurse tells me your blood pressure is a little up. Anything been different, any reason for that that you know of?"

"Nosir."

"I see. Have you been able to take the blood pressure medicines I gave you last time?"

"Yessir," she says.

I leaf through the few pages in the chart and notice it has been six months since the last visit, when I started her on a new blood pressure medicine, gave her a month's supply, and asked her to come back within a week. "Hmm," I begin, not knowing quite how to reconcile the discrepancy. "I wonder how you could have had enough pills to last you all this time. I just gave you enough for a month last time. Did you get a prescription somewhere else?"

"Nosir."

"Did you take a pill every day, the way we talked about?"

"Yessir."

I'm at a loss. I try another tack. "Is there something wrong with the pills? Are there any side effects that bother you? Did you have to stop the pills for some reason?"

"Nosir. I took a pill every day."

"But I only gave you enough for a month. Where did you get enough to last you six months?"

Silence. Ms. Dixon continues to stare at the floor.

"Is there anything I can do that would make it easier for you to get in here for medicines or for appointments?"

Silence.

We start again. Because her blood pressure is so high and potentially dangerous, I give her a quick-acting medication, but her pressure falls only a little, to 210/130. I consider sending her to the emergency room for treatment, but I've already tried that (three times with her and numerous times in similar situations with other patients), always with distressingly similar results: Either she doesn't go to the emergency room at all and drops completely out of sight (the most common response), or she does go and the blood pressure is brought down out of the danger range, although nowhere near normal. Then the emergency room doctor (probably assuming that she's been taking her medications as she says she has and that they aren't working) changes her regimen around, gives her prescriptions she can't afford to fill, and tells her to come back to the hospital medical clinic in a week ... which she won't do. Instead she goes home, and within forty-eight hours her blood pressure is back up to 220/140, where it remains until—"feeling poorly"—she returns to our office one or two or three or more months later, now supposedly on a different regimen of pills the names of which she never learned.

I decide to give Ms. Dixon enough medication for a week and ask her if she can return tomorrow afternoon (knowing full well that if she has a stroke tonight, I will—in the eyes of most medical professionals and all legal ones—be grossly negligent for not having sent her to the emergency room). She agrees; but the next afternoon, of course, she doesn't show up. As sometimes happens, however, several other people are also no-shows, so the waiting room is empty. I decide, as I do from time to time, to make a home visit. Perhaps in her home I will be able to understand her situation a little better. Ms. Dixon has no phone, so we can't call ahead, but she lives on the next block. Robert Davids, a nurse/handyman who volunteers many hours a week at Community of Hope in addition to his forty-hour job at a local hospital, accompanies me, because the building in which Ms. Dixon lives has a reputation for toughness.

About a dozen or so young black men are slouching around the entrance to the old brick building. More are moving in the shadows just inside the door. The scent of marijuana as well as an exotic odor I don't recognize hangs heavy in the air, and money is changing hands. The group parts reluctantly, and I'm very aware of Robert's and my white skin as we brush against the boys, who seem to stand deliberately in our way. Once out of the bright sunlight, our eyes take a few seconds to adjust, for there are no lights in the dark hallways. We proceed cautiously toward the stairs. The hall on the far side of the stairwell is apparently unused, for it is entirely filled with trash; an old refrigerator, its door dangling crookedly on broken hinges, is tipped against the wall. Every single window in the stairwell has been broken. As we ascend to the second floor, I notice that the doors to many apartments have been ripped off. Gradually it dawns on me: The building is abandoned. No one could be living here.

With considerable trepidation Robert and I climb to the third floor, although there seems little possibility of finding anyone. There is no railing on the stairs, and I hug the wall in the darkness. This landing, too, is jammed with trash, its windows broken. We grope our way down the hall in pitch darkness. Light filters out from around the edges of a few doors, but most are dark.

I can't see apartment numbers at all. My heart is pounding, and I wonder what I'm doing here. Could I suddenly fall through some unseen hole in the floor? Will a drug addict, desperate for cash and lurking in this dark hallway, jump me? In this blackness I'm suddenly, painfully, aware of my whiteness and of how little I belong here. Will we have any trouble making it past that gang of young men on our way out? It is hard to believe that our well-lit and friendly clinic is less than fifty yards away.

I literally have to feel for the numbers on the doors. Fortunately "342," the number Ms. Dixon gave us, is the third one we come to. I knock. No one answers. I knock again, more tentatively, hoping, perhaps, that there will be no answer, but the door now opens about five inches. A sliver of a young boy's face appears in the crack.

"Hello, I'm Dr. Hilfiker. Is Ms. Dixon at home?"

"Who?"

"Ms. Dixon?"

"Oh," the face disappears for a second, leaving only

small hands holding the edge of the door. I hear the muffled
sound of voices back there somewhere. The face reappears,
the door opened a little wider this time. "She ain't home."
"Well, do you know when she might be back?"
"No."
A little girl of perhaps four has wandered up behind the
boy to watch. I glance into the apartment and past the girl.
As far as I can see, there is—except for a plain kitchen ta-
ble offering jelly and bread—neither furniture nor a rug. A
single, bare lightbulb hangs from the ceiling.
"Is there anyone else home whom I could talk to?"
There is a split-second pause as the boy glances some-
where behind the door. "No," he then says quickly.
"Well, could you take a message for me?"
The boy says nothing. "Please ask your mom to call Dr.
Hilfiker at the clinic. Dr. *Hil-fi-ker.*"
He shuts the door before I can offer to write anything
down. I can hear the drunken voices of adults rising in the
background, but I can't tell for sure whether they come
from Ms. Dixon's apartment or one nearby. I don't stop to
check it out.
We find our way down and push our way through the
dope and money changing hands at the building's entrance.
Suddenly we are out in the sunlight, very far from the darkness and despair we have just witnessed.
I have seen Ms. Dixon only once or twice since, and I
have not gone back to look for her.
It is easy to imagine that Marjawn Dixon finds compliance with my suggestions impossible. There is a kind of
chaos here, a chaos that burdens the lives of many of the
poor, inhibiting them from accomplishing—or perhaps even
considering—things that the rest of us take for granted. Ms.
Dixon has much weightier things on her mind than her
blood pressure or her appointment with me. And what am
I to do about her? Nothing, I suppose. But it is hard to
stand by and do nothing, especially when I think of those
children alone in that apartment. And it is hard to accept
my own powerlessness. I'm the doctor, yet far from being

able to cure everything, here I have a patient who desperately needs my help—and I find I can't do anything. The ability to withstand such overwhelming chaos, to work within it, to make decisions in spite of it, is a practical discipline the doctor must acquire quickly if he is to survive the inner city. And just as difficult as the chaos without is the uncertainty within—so contrary to medicine's promise of a rational methodology—with which the poverty doctor must also come to terms. It may be this willingness to stay with my patients regardless of the vast uncertainty, and to accept the resulting intensification of my own inner chaos, that best defines my work.

Eugenia Delp is in her fifties, overweight, with many medical problems, but she is usually an effusive, bubbly person. On this day she's rather quiet. I ask her what brings her to the office, and we begin talking about her high blood pressure. Eugenia does not like coming to the clinic, and I am a little surprised that she has voluntarily appeared to talk about her blood pressure when it is really no worse than it has been in the several years I've cared for her. But I am hopeful that perhaps she is taking a little more responsibility for her health. We talk for a few minutes, and I fill out a new prescription. I ask her how she's feeling, and she says that things are okay.

As she leaves the office, I again find myself a little puzzled by her visit; nothing of importance came up. A week later I learn that Eugenia is in the hospital. Several days after I saw her, apparently, she went by ambulance to a hospital emergency room and was admitted for heart failure. Her daughters have wondered aloud to Lois Wagner, the director of the Health Services, why I didn't discover the problem on her visit to the office. Eugenia had reported to them that I'd given her a clean bill of health.

I am chagrined, and—my memory being what it is—I pull out her chart to remind myself of what occurred. As far as I can reconstruct matters, Eugenia came to the office feeling quite sick but never actually put her symptoms into words.

Did she assume that her presence in the office was complaint enough, that it was then *my* job to ask the questions that would clarify her illness? It is not only among the poor that physicians find people who seem to believe the doctor is capable of seeing through them and into their health, as long as they present their bodies for inspection; but such beliefs seem especially common here in the inner city. Perhaps she felt that—having come to my office—she'd done her part.

Or had I cowed her into silence with my questions? Perhaps I assumed too quickly that she was there just to follow up on her high blood pressure. Perhaps she, reasonably enough, interpreted my questions to mean that I was only interested in her pressure. Perhaps my expressions of concern over her pressure—which never quite gets down to normal—were so threatening to her at that moment that her own complaints slid into insignificance.

Or did I make such a big deal about the blood pressure that she felt guilty, unable to complain about other symptoms without feeling even more of a failure? For some people who experience daily degradation, "saving face" has a very high value, and they might sooner return home sick than once again expose their "failures." Especially in the ghetto, where abuse and lack of success are daily realities, the doctor must explore the details of a person's life with extreme sensitivity. Had I neglected to do so?

Or perhaps Eugenia had, in fact, told me about her symptoms, and I had simply disregarded them. Perhaps she had complained of "tiredness" or "stress" and I mistakenly tuned out her complaints, thinking them to reflect only her emotional state or the imposed stress of her difficult life. Some days, virtually all my patients are "tired," and—after considering the common causes—I can't bring myself to look thoroughly for the exotic physical illness that, in rare instances, may be causing their fatigue. Had I failed to pick

up on certain clues she gave me? Exactly what happened
will undoubtedly never be clear. Part of the frustration a doctor in my situation faces is
never really learning from his mistakes. Because the social
and emotional issues are so complex; because specialists
can rarely help with the kinds of difficulties that trouble my
patients; because my patients and I can seldom sit down
and discuss our difficulties in understanding one another
(for even that discussion requires us to share common assumptions); because people who get better don't usually
come back for follow-up and those who don't get better often go to an emergency room—because of all these factors,
I don't get the kind of feedback about my mistakes that is
necessary if I am to learn from them. What can I learn from
Mrs. Delp? To be "more careful"? What can I do differently next time? I don't know, and I have discovered no
way of finding out. There is rarely a resolution to this tension. I must simply give myself permission to live in a
great deal of chaos.

The practice of poverty medicine often takes place in the
absence of shared assumptions, which only increases the
disorder and uncertainty. To my patients my questions must
often seem unrelated to their primary concerns, while the
history of their symptoms—easily the most important part
of any evaluation—remains a mystery to me. When I am
trying, for instance, to determine the likelihood of pregnancy or the significance of vaginal bleeding, I frequently
ask a woman the date of her last menstrual period. The in-
variable answer is either "This month" or "Last month."
When I ask her to be more precise, she often seems confused by my question. It's not really a matter of memory;
my inquiry seems senseless to her. For many of the women
in my practice, menstrual cycles are bound to the calendar
months rather than to a cycle of so many weeks and days.
A woman will sometimes come to the office worried because "my period came twice this month," by which she
means that the first menstrual period began on January 2

and the next on January 30. She will then be concerned because she "misses a period" during February. This simple difference in the way we understand things can usually be compensated for, but there are other, more complex gaps in communication that leave my patients feeling ignored or misunderstood.

Trust—that crucial ingredient between physician and patient—is often lacking in the sort of medicine I now practice. I want to make sure, for instance, that Tajuana Billins, a fifteen-year-old girl with symptoms of a serious pelvic infection, does not have a pregnancy in her fallopian tubes (a so-called ectopic pregnancy, which doctors sometimes mistake for a pelvic infection). I explain that we must determine whether she is pregnant and I ask her about her last menstrual period and her most recent episode of sexual intercourse. She tells me that her period came "last month," but assures me that she has not had sex in over two months. Several minutes later, examining a specimen of her vaginal fluid under the microscope to check for venereal disease, I see sperm vigorously moving about. I return to ask again about her history of intercourse, and she resolutely asserts that she has not had intercourse in over two months, a story she sticks to even after I reemphasize the importance of the question.

Why is she lying to me? Perhaps, for reasons that I don't begin to understand, her story isn't a lie to her. Perhaps talking about sex to a male, especially a white male, is worse than lying. Perhaps in her mind the consequences of opening the door to her personal life, even a crack, are too dire. Perhaps an overly strict or abusive home environment has made hiding her personal life a necessity. Perhaps it is just adolescence. A lot of possible explanations flood my mind, but are any of them correct? In the end, I go with my gut instinct (not always right, either): I decide against confronting her with what is so obviously untrue. I do not blame Tajuana; but our inability to communicate effectively, whatever the cause, leaves me with little reliable information on which to base either a diagnosis or a relationship.

In my Minnesota practice as well, of course, I was sometimes told incomplete or false stories. But my patient and I generally shared a common language, so that someone who did not want to reveal everything to me could nonetheless communicate her reluctance, and I could at least recognize the gaps in my own understanding. Or—when caught in an outright lie—a patient could find a way to backtrack, to give me enough of the truth to get me off her case.

Tajuana and I, however, speak such different languages that I'm far from certain about the real nature of her disease. I know there is something else wrong, something going on behind the presenting complaint, but here—unlike in my middle-class clinic—my intuition is of minimal value. Because my patients and I face each other across barriers of culture and language, I usually cannot "get inside" their heads to find out what is wrong.

It is not possible to discuss poverty medicine without talking about yet another formidable barrier—that of racial difference. While in absolute numbers most poor people in our country are white, African Americans and Hispanics are three times more likely than whites to be poor, and the inner-city patient is likely to be a person of color. Yet poverty medicine—at least in urban areas—is largely practiced by white professionals. In medicine, as in so many other areas of American life, the person with power is still white; the person needing help, black or Hispanic.

In the 1960s, in the days of Black Power, a white physician practicing in a black neighborhood might have been asked by black people what he was doing there, why he wasn't fighting racism in his own environment. But thirty years later certain dreams have died. No black person has ever said to me directly or, as far as I can remember, even implied that I don't belong on Belmont Street. The reason, I think, is obvious, the reality as clear as it is lamentable: If the white doctors and nurses and lawyers leave Belmont Street, no one will replace us. White theorists and organizers will, from time to time, accuse us of disempowering the people with whom we work, but until those critics show me how I can practice without disempowering my patients or where my patients will receive good medical care when I leave, I find it hard to justify departure.

But despite my pragmatic response to these issues, a problem persists. American history is often read as a long legacy of white people telling black people what to do; and the work of the inner-city doctor can seem like just another instance of this unequal dynamic. White people have historically exploited black communities—have come in, taken the money, and left. The poor inner-city black person has reason to see the white inner-city doctor as someone who comes into the community and earns handsome fees (even my "austerity salary" at Community of Hope is three times what many of my patients earn working full-time), while his patients haven't enough to pay the rent. I live at Christ House, but "upstairs," where the patients never go; I live "in" the community, but not directly on Belmont Street. The history of American social reform is filled with white people "helping" black people by "doing for" them. The medical model itself, in which the doctor does *for* and does *to* the patient, is an inherently disempowering one.

So the white doctor of poverty medicine practices within a deeply troubled historical context. How do I deal with the sneaking suspicions (which I, on bad days, share) that I am—despite my best intentions—exploiting my patients? Racial prejudice is so thoroughly ingrained that no one of us—black or white—can be free of the charge of "racism." The best we can do is acknowledge racism, try to understand it, and move on.

These reflections inevitably return me to the same questions: What am I doing here? What can I offer my patients? If I do so little good by traditional medical standards, if my very presence may be disempowering, what *can* I do? Ultimately, the answer is the same one every good doctor anywhere must come to: I can offer myself and my presence as a healer. The recent tide of technological medicine has tended to erode our understanding of the fundamental imperative for any physician—to be a healing presence. Because our antibiotics and our CAT scans and our heart transplants promise such power, we risk confusing the use of those tools with the most basic task of doctoring: to understand, to comfort, to encourage, to *be with* the patient in his or her distress.

With its potentially distracting techniques and technology, traditional medicine may *need* poverty medicine as a reminder that the primary role of the good physician is to offer unconditional acceptance of the patient's being; to clarify (without judging) the cause of the illness; to honor the pain, to recognize the fear, and to hold on to hope.

Chapter 12

CLINT WOODER

I can't recall Clint Wooder's actual arrival at Christ House. He was one of many middle-aged, severely alcoholic, homeless men admitted directly from the hospital. Records remind me he was probably the worst alcoholic I'd seen in the course of my work in the city. His liver had been devastated by years of drinking, and as is often the result, his abdomen was distended by a massive amount of fluid. This time he'd been hospitalized after vomiting blood and treated for bleeding veins around the base of his esophagus. There hadn't been much to do for his cirrhosis except wait to see if the fluid in his abdomen would be reabsorbed with abstinence from alcohol, rest, and a decent diet. He was lucky to be alive, although I doubt he felt very lucky at the time.

Like our other residents, he probably lay low during his first days at Christ House, trying to figure out just what our angle was. It would have been typical for him to stay close to his bed, leaving his room only for the dining room downstairs, where he would heap up huge plates of food (not quite trusting that there would be a next meal), trying to remain inconspicuous among the thirty-three other homeless men recovering from their own afflictions.

The first I remember of him was an examination some weeks later. Clint was a white man about my own age, born in the hills of Kentucky. He was tall, big, and—except for the soft bulge of the abdomen—an angular man. His face was scarred from previous battles, his eyes were penetrating, his voice held a muted twang. When he undressed, the contrast between the dark skin on his face and hands, roughened by years on the streets, and the pasty white of his trunk and legs was startling. The skin over his abdomen, stretched thin, was unnaturally shiny, almost translucent, a reminder of the inexorable illness below. Clint was different from many of the others I'd worked with: He didn't avert his eyes. I felt he was incapable of lying.

"Doc, I got no control over alcohol. I can only hope I won't drink today 'cause it's too much to think about tomorrow, too. They said in the hospital my liver was shot, an' I guess it is, an' I know what it's from. Said I almost died. I got another chance, I guess, and I'm sober . . . at least right now. I just pray to my Higher Power I can stay sober until tonight."

And he would smile—a hearty smile in spite of the stained and missing teeth—and glance down at the floor and back at me, and then he'd laugh and immediately try to cover it up as if it weren't quite right. I was drawn in, trusted.

Clint not only went to the four required Alcoholics Anonymous meetings held weekly at Christ House, but he also sought out as many other AA meetings as he could, anywhere he could find them. "How many meetings do you go to?" I once asked him.

He looked at me with that grin, glanced at the floor, and laughed. "Yesterday I went to four, an' I took the bus down to the Metropolis Club this mornin'. I can just catch the bus back to the church for the noon meetin' there. And then the one here this afternoon." He looked at me and, I suppose, saw the puzzlement on my face.

"Doc, I'm just a drunk an' I gotta go to meetin's all day long. I can't promise you I won't drink, 'cause I prob'ly will. I just live from day to day, hopin' I won't drink today. I can't even guarantee you that! Someday I'll just be walkin' down the street, and someone'll hand me a bottle, and I'll start drinkin' for no reason at all; an' I won't stop until they carry me into the hospital. Twice now the doctors told me the next time it was gonna be the morgue. I suppose it is."

I tried to imagine what it would be like to live so close to the edge, to see my self-destruction so clearly, and to experience so profoundly my life's dependence on my own wobbly balance. I knew, by now, that we are all in some sense like Clint, all sometimes powerless before our urges, and that our illusions of control can crack in an instant. But when a person like me leans out over the abyss, it is with a safety harness around his waist and wide nets below. For Clint there was nothing between him and the void, and he knew it. Clint had profound respect for the abyss.

I was Clint's physician. I had become something like his counselor, giving him not so much medical advice as a chance to talk about himself. By profession I was his guide as he dealt with his illness and his explosive feelings, but I was guiding him over territory I had never experienced, could never experience, myself. From the safety of my own situation, I could watch and nod reassuringly, offering advice, but never really understanding what it must be to live like that. I felt honored by his trust.

Clint stayed dry. I thought, in fact, that he had it made. After a few months' physical recovery in Christ House, he moved into one of the Samaritan Inns. The Inns, however, are closed to the men during the day, so Clint continued to eat at Christ House and volunteered there as a handyman. He became something of a fixture downstairs, always willing to help out, always ready to take on or create new jobs for himself. One thing was clear to him: He had to keep busy.

Clint was concerned about his health and, unlike most of the men, kept his weekly medical appointments with me. He told me a little of his past, and we would talk occasionally about his dreams: to keep a job, to support himself, to have a place of his own. I found myself fascinated by him, attracted to him, cheering for him in his recovery. Although he had been sober for six months, Clint was also—as was evident in our sessions—gradually growing more restless and agitated. He began to complain with increasing bitterness: "They don't give me enough to do. I can't just sit around or I get The Angry. Sister Marcella, she's watchin' me, just waitin' for me to do somethin' wrong so she can throw me out. She says she don't like guys from Samaritan Inns here all the time, but she's lookin' right at me. An' Miller better watch his step, how he talks to me.

"I know what it is," he'd say as we sat in the little exam room off the downstairs hall. "It happens every time. I get The Angry. Every time I get sober for a while, The Angry comes, an' I have to start drinkin' agin. If I drink, it goes away an' I ain't got The Angry no more. It's only when I'm sober. An' there's no way I can control it. You gotta do somethin', Doc, give me somethin' to take or somethin' to do, or I'm gonna hurt somebody. Or else I'm gonna start drinkin' agin." And he would stand and pace the room like the panther a few blocks away at the National Zoo.

I began to be afraid for him. I did not believe Clint would become violent with me, but I could see his agitation, and I now took seriously his earlier protestations that he was "just a drunk."

He knew more about himself than I had realized. He understood that his rage went way back to those years after his father died (Clint was two) when he was reared by an older, alcoholic brother who beat him regularly. As a small child Clint could not protect himself, and apparently no one intervened. I found it hard to believe his claim that he started drinking at age five, but he insisted he learned early to douse his feelings with alcohol. He'd been drinking ever since. Sober, he tried to contain the cauldron of feelings inside, roiling, about to boil over. When the feelings became too much, he would batter himself with intoxication, almost killing himself—and thus, paradoxically, relieve his rage.

His abused childhood left Clint with unfathomed psychological chaos, and he needed help. I'm not a psychiatrist or psychologist, so at our sessions I mostly listened, not pretending to do anything medical but offering Clint a sympathetic ear. I became quickly aware, however, that his emotional tumult demanded more than my sympathy. "Clint, you're right. The Angry is going to take you under. We can both see it coming, and I can't seem to do much to help you. Would you be willing to go see a counselor or a therapist and spend some time talking with him? Maybe he could find some way to help."

"You mean a shrink?" His face clouded, then hardened with determination. "Hell, I'll talk with anybody. I gotta do somethin'! Maybe he can give me somethin' for this."

But I could find no private psychiatrist willing even to see Clint for an initial evaluation, much less work for months with a homeless alcoholic who could pay nothing. In desperation—knowing only too well how little we could expect—I turned to the public clinics.

I called a psychiatrist I knew in the city's mental health system and lobbied for Clint. My colleague assured me that he knew the best psychiatrist-in-training in Washington (much of the public psychiatric care here is provided by doctors-in-training) and that he would arrange an appointment for Clint. A week later a young psychiatric resident did call me to schedule Clint's initial interview. I was relieved. I was off the hook for a while.

"It was okay," Clint said in response to my question at our next meeting. "That doctor seemed okay, the psychiatrist. I kinda liked talkin' to him." He paused and looked at me; he got up from his chair and started pacing back and forth. "But we didn't do nothin' about The Angry," he said darkly. "An' I don't know if I can last until the next one."

"What do you mean, 'last'?" I said.

"He said he could only see me for twenty minutes every two weeks."

Twenty minutes! There had to be some mistake. What

could twenty minutes of psychotherapy every two weeks accomplish for a person like Clint?

After several days of intermittent and unsuccessful calls, I finally managed to reach the resident by phone—not an easy trick within the city's bureaucracy. But there was no mistake. Twenty minutes was the most he could offer an outpatient who was not actively psychotic. "I know it's not enough," he said with some sympathy in his voice. "But it's all I'm allowed with the mental health patients. I see most of my patients once a month. I think Clint needs lots of help, so I managed to get him on the schedule every two weeks. But if you could find somebody who could see him more often, he really needs something like that. Maybe you could try a little Haldol; that sometimes gives people like him some relief."

We tried the Haldol—a major tranquilizer, it succeeded only in sedating Clint—but Clint had gotten the message: There was no one to help him. A week or two later, while I was at the clinic, I received a phone call from Christ House. At lunch, Clint had gotten into an argument and—in response to a resident's abusive language—had grabbed him by the neck, choking him. A staff person tried to intervene, and Clint went after him with a crutch. Clint knew we would not tolerate violence. He had done what he needed to do to get himself barred from Christ House.

The next morning, a Saturday, I didn't know what to expect as I walked over to the Samaritan Inn to confront him. I had never seen Clint's anger, only traces of it beneath the surface. "Whadda you want?" he said as he opened the door. "You gonna kick me outta here?" There was no grin this time, no laugh.

I sank down in a chair. "*I'm* not going to," I said. "I don't work over here. But the staff here's probably going to."

"I know," he said.

"Clint, what happened over there? You knew you couldn't do that. Why'd you blow it?"

"We had some words," he replied, almost meekly, "and I grabbed him, that's all."

We looked at each other. This was the same person I'd met with every week for four months. I couldn't imagine him trying to strangle anyone. "Marcella said you did more than grab him. She said you choked him. She was afraid you'd kill him."

"I told you I just grabbed him!" I watched a fire light in his eyes, something new, something frightening. Clint stood up. "I'm going to kill that son of a bitch. He can hide over there at Christ House, but he'll have to come out on the streets sometime, walk by an alley—an' I'll kill him." He looked at me with defiance. This was "The Angry," a rageful stranger. Within a minute or so I could recognize Clint again, but The Angry was close upon him.

I was scared for Clint and I was scared for others. If he could try to strangle someone in the security of the dining room at Christ House, there was no telling what would happen on the streets. I searched my mind furiously. The only alternative I could imagine to Clint's quick return to the streets and premature death was psychiatric hospitalization.

But when I proposed this, Clint's body stiffened and his hands clenched. He looked me dead in the eye with an expression somewhere between rage and helplessness. "I been there once before," he said, and then pronounced every word with emphasis: *"An' I ain't never goin' back there agin.* You understand? Never!"

I understood his resolve, but I needed to understand more. "Where were you, Clint? What did they put you in the hospital for?"

"That place over there across the river, where Hinckley's at. It was the same thing, The Angry, but what they do to you there, I ain't never goin' back again."

I retreated, desperately; I was in way over my head, and there was no one to help. "Clint, St. Elizabeth's isn't the only option. Lots of the other hospitals have psychiatric units, and you could go to one of them. I know those places, and they're good places. They'll help you. Clint, I'm afraid for you. Won't you come with me?"

I could watch Clint struggle with my suggestion, trying to choose between his tenuous trust in me and his fear of "that place." I wasn't being completely honest: I didn't have personal experience with the hospital psychiatric units, and I wasn't sure they would be better than St. Elizabeth's. But I thought that Clint would have a better chance at a private hospital than he would at St. E.'s.

I left unsaid the threat of involuntary commitment, partly because I didn't know how I'd pull it off. I'd learned that systems have a way of not working when dealing with the poor. I was flying by the seat of my pants in this strange situation, but I knew intuitively that it was important for Clint to feel as much control as he could under the circumstances.

Clint finally consented. "I'll go any place you want me to go, as long as it's not St. E.'s. I ain't goin' to that place." I called to make sure there was a bed available in the psych unit of one of the best hospitals in the city and drove Clint there.

The check-in at the emergency room desk was brief, and Clint was interviewed promptly, in stark contrast to the six- to eight-hour waits at hospitals in the poor sections of town. Dr. Lilliwen, a first-year psychiatric resident, saw Clint and interviewed me briefly as well. She agreed Clint needed hospitalization to protect himself and others from his rage. She left to make arrangements, only to return in ten minutes. There were no beds available, she informed me.

"No," I said, reflexively, as if to correct her, and I could hear my voice breaking. "I called less than two hours ago, and I was told there would be no problems with bed space. It's now nine A.M. Do you mean you filled those empty beds between seven and nine on a Saturday morning?"

Dr. Lilliwen, a pleasant young woman, looked flustered. "I'm not sure what you were told this morning," she said evasively, "but there's no room for Mr. Wooder in the unit now. Besides, the attending psychiatrist is worried about his violence. We're not a locked unit." Something had happened in the ten minutes since the resident had left us fully intending to admit Clint. Perhaps it was Clint's status as a Medicaid patient, which meant the hospital would not get its usual reimbursement. Perhaps it was Clint's status as a homeless alcoholic, which would disturb this middle-class hospital's psychiatric unit. Perhaps it was the attending psychiatrist's discomfort with the potential violence, although this was an issue that a city hospital must face every day. I didn't know for sure what it was, but I was pretty sure the refusal had something to do with Clint's poverty. Whatever it was, the decision had been made someplace higher up the ladder than this first-year resident, and she had no power to change it. I just stood there.

"They said there was no bed for him on the floor," Dr. Lilliwen said uncomfortably. "Let me see if I can't find someplace else that will take him." For the next three hours Clint waited in a tiny cubicle while I shuttled back and forth between Dr. Lilliwen, who was searching in vain for another hospital, and Clint, who was becoming increasingly agitated. Finally, it was clear: There was not a single private hospital in Washington willing to admit Clint Wooder to its psychiatric unit, even though he was one of the lucky ones on the streets with full-coverage Medicaid. The only remaining option was St. Elizabeth's. I went back to the little room to break the news.

He interrupted me in mid-sentence, stood up, turned his back on me, and deliberately put on his jacket. "No way! I told you I'd go anyplace else you wanted, but not to that place. That's just for crazy people, an' I ain't crazy. You don't know what they do to you in there." He was no longer willing to look at me.

"But, Clint, you know you need help or you're going to hurt somebody. You told me that yourself. And you know what will happen if you really hurt somebody. Prison or the morgue will be a lot worse than St. E.'s. C'mon, you won't have to stay in there long. We've got to get you some help."

"No way!" The answer was always the same. Clint remained standing, his jacket on. The longer we talked, the more agitated he became. Suddenly he turned and stalked out of the hospital. I trailed him like a pleading child, struggling to keep up with his long stride, struggling to reason with him. It was no use. Emotionally exhausted, I stopped on the sidewalk and watched him walk away. I retraced my steps into the hospital.

Hanging unspoken over our interactions ever since Clint's assault the day before had been the issue of involuntary commitment. As a licensed physician caring for a patient who is "a danger to himself or to others," I have the legal right (and responsibility) to initiate commitment proceedings by filling out papers that direct the police to bring the patient in, willing or not, to be examined by an independent psychiatrist. In the District of Columbia, that is usually done by the psychiatrists at St. Elizabeth's. If the public psychiatrist agrees that the patient is indeed a danger to self or others, the patient is kept in the psychiatric hospital until a formal legal hearing before a judge (which must take place within seventy-two hours), at which time a final decision is made about whether the patient will be forced to accept psychiatric care.

I was ambivalent. The trained physician in me believed Clint needed to be in the hospital any way we could get him there, even if commitment was necessary. The poverty doctor in me knew how alone I was in this: For practical purposes, I was the only professional available to Clint, and I had nothing else left in my bag of tricks to offer him but the terrors of St. E.'s. If I couldn't get Clint into a hospital, I was going to be stuck with a situation I couldn't manage. The friend-of-Clint in me, however, was not so sure that commitment would ultimately help Clint. I knew The Angry well enough to know that Clint was unlikely ever to respond to forced help.

I had mentioned commitment to Dr. Lilliwen when we

first came to the private hospital, hoping it would not be necessary. Now that Clint had walked out, she raised the issue again, and I reluctantly agreed it would be a good idea. Feeling frustrated with my powerlessness—and frustrated with wasting what was to have been my weekend off—I ignored my discomfort in abandoning Clint to emergency room doctors who hardly knew him. I was only too happy, in fact, to bow out and allow the commitment to proceed through the private hospital. It would, I told myself, be shorter (the preadmission evaluation could be performed in *any* hospital), easier (similar commitments passed through this emergency room regularly), and more likely to succeed (my experiences with John Turnell and others had not given me great confidence that I would be able to orchestrate the entire process successfully). Dr. Lilliwen called the attending psychiatrist, who gave the order to notify the police to find Clint for forcible commitment to St. Elizabeth's Hospital.

Clint, not surprisingly, was nowhere to be found.

But Clint *did* return to the Samaritan Inn that Saturday night. The staff person on duty called Dr. Lilliwen, who—to my amazement—was able to convince Clint over the phone to come back to the emergency room. There he was forcibly restrained and involuntarily committed to St. Elizabeth's. About eleven that evening Dr. Lilliwen called me to report that Clint was on his way to St. E.'s. I received the news with conflicting feelings. Relieved that Clint was finally safe in a hospital, I also felt that I'd betrayed him in handing him over to the system. Even though I had, technically, kept my hands clean, I knew that the involuntary commitment would damage whatever trust had built up between us. Reassured that he was at least physically secure, however, I prepared to relax for the rest of my "weekend off."

But come Sunday morning, I received a call from the social worker at Samaritan Inns. Clint was no longer at St. E.'s. Without consulting with the referring psychiatric staff at the private hospital, with me, or with any of the readily available eyewitnesses to Clint's violence, St. Elizabeth's admitting psychiatrist had determined in a short interview late at night that Clint was a danger neither to himself nor to others. At three o'clock that morning, less than six hours after his transfer, Clint had been released to the streets without any of those who had been working intensively with him even being notified.

I was angry about having wasted a Saturday off, guilty for bowing out at the last minute, depressed at Clint's utter lack of options, enraged that the "system" would simply spew Clint back onto the streets without the help he so desperately needed and wanted—and I was in despair that all this had happened at the expense of my relationship with Clint. A bed would, of course, have been available in the private psychiatric unit if Clint had been alcoholic, destructive, and affluent. How quickly would a middle-class person complaining of uncontrollable rage after assaulting someone be hospitalized, or at least provided with intensive care? Once again, the system had abandoned a poor person—one, in this case, willing to be helped.

I, too, felt abandoned. The system had not been there to help me, either, as I struggled to handle this problem so much bigger than myself. I, too, felt hopeless about Clint's ultimately conquering his alcoholism. The anger I was experiencing was not just vicarious. Though I didn't know quite whom to be angry at, I *was* angry. My desire to be with and help this indigent alcoholic had subjected me to some of the same forces that buffeted him.

Amazingly, Clint did not return immediately to the bottle. Although we had barred him from Christ House because of the assault, Samaritan Inns decided to allow him to stay there, and he continued to meet with me for several weeks. But something had indeed been lost. Clint had retreated into himself. He started to miss his appointments, and when he came, he was sullen and resentful. One day, Clint disappeared. Then came word that he was on the streets and drinking again.

Two weeks later Barbara Ryan, an aide at Christ House,

noticed Clint on Connecticut Avenue, drunk and disheveled. She called me at the office and then persuaded Clint to travel across the city with her to Community of Hope, where she sat with him until I could examine him.

I was rushing from one exam room to another when I first saw the huddled shape. I could tell it was a man, but— even expecting Clint—I didn't recognize him and continued with my scheduled patients. Later, I looked out into the waiting area. I noticed Barbara, and there was an older white man sitting next to her in the corner, his tall body slumped in a chair, hidden in a large, dirty coat. His face and hands were olive green, a skin color I had never seen before! His features were startlingly distorted.

I led Clint into the exam room. He was drunk and sullen; the energy in those eyes had been replaced by a vacant stare.

I could think of only one thing to offer. "Clint, would you be willing to go down to detox?"

He shook his head dully, his eyes never leaving the floor. "It won't do no good. No one can help me. I'll drink 'til I die. Besides, they won't let me in down there." His voice was flat, emotionless.

"They've got to let you in," I said. "That's what they're there for. It's public detox. They're not *allowed* to turn anyone away."

"They won't let me in."

"I'll take you down. Will you let me take you to detox, Clint?"

He was silent a minute, not meeting my gaze. "Yeah . . . but you'll see, they won't let me in."

Office hours were essentially over. I biked back to Christ House to pick up the house van and returned for Clint, half-expecting him to be gone. But he was still there, sagging into the chair in the now-empty waiting room. He moved slowly, stiffly into the van like a frail old man, and we drove silently. Halfway across the city, while we were stopped at a light, I noticed his hand moving toward the door handle. But he hesitated, then relaxed into the seat. Some part of him wanted to stay alive.

I walked behind Clint as he led me up the steps of the nondescript brick building that housed the detox unit on the sprawling grounds of D.C. General Hospital. He knew his way, which was fortunate, for there were no signs indicating what the building might be or through which of its several doors we should enter. Clint went right to the middle doors, however, and pushed a button. We waited a long time for a guard to open it and lead us through two large, high-ceilinged, absolutely barren rooms, echoing our silence like the empty anterooms in an old European castle where the once-rich count and his family huddle in three small rooms upstairs. The guard led us to the second floor, to what I took to be the receiving station. Clint, quite familiar with the routine, slumped onto the bench opposite the desk. As we waited, an occasional middle-aged black man in pajamas moved wearily in one direction or the other down the bare, dimly lit hall. The reek of stale cigarette smoke hung in the air. Impatient, I stopped the first person I saw in street clothes. "I've brought a man for admission," I said. "Who do I see?"

"What's his name?" he asked.

"Clint Wooder."

"Name sounds familiar." He looked down at Clint's slumping body. "Oh, yeah. Wooder." He turned back to me. "Ain't no reason to have him here. He'll walk out as soon as you leave. He signed out before, he'll sign out again."

He turned and addressed himself to Clint, raising his voice. "You signed out last time, Wooder. A.M.A.! You know what that means? Against Medical Advice! You gonna sign out again? What you come down here for? You know you ain't gonna give up drinkin'. What you botherin' us for?" Clint made no response.

I decided to ignore the attendant's hostility and asked for the person in charge of admission. He nodded toward a well-dressed man in his forties who was walking by. I be-

gan to explain my mission. He cut me short and led me into
a cramped office.

"I'm Dr. Hilfiker," I said, hoping that the title might
count for something. "From Christ House . . . ?" He seemed
not to hear. "I've been working with Mr. Wooder for over
six months now, but he started drinking two weeks ago. I'd
like to leave him here for detox. We'll take him back to
Christ House when the three days are up."

"If he wants to stay, we'll take him. We can't force nobody to stay, you know. If he wants to stay, we'll take
him."

I went out and asked Clint again, afraid that the verbal
abuse from the first attendant had already taken its toll.
"Yeah, I'll stay," Clint said angrily. "I told you I'd stay, and
I'll stay."

Relieved, I was on my way out of the building when a
third attendant came walking out with Clint's old chart.
"You'd better come back and talk with Mr. Moore," he said
to me. "Wooder signed out A.M.A. a year ago last January.
He can't stay here."

I was led back again to the second attendant, Mr. Moore,
who began flipping through Clint's old chart. "Yeah, I remember him now. You might as well take him. Wooder's
not gonna stay here."

"He said he'd stay."

"He won't stay," Mr. Moore said laconically. As if to
prove his point, Mr. Moore walked out to the bench across
from the door. "Sit up, Wooder," he demanded in a loud
voice. "You wanna stay here? You left before. You gonna
stay here this time?" The tone was belligerent, aggressive.
"You know how long you got to stay here? You sure you
wanna stay here?"

Clint looked up, and some of the fire was back in his
eyes. "Yeah, I know how long I got to stay here. Seventy-
two hours." He virtually barked the words, his voice angry
yet somehow beaten. *He* knew what was coming.

"You *sure* you want to stay here?"

Clint stood up, his hands stuffed in the oversize coat. I

was afraid he was going to start swinging. "Well, if you don't want me, I'll go." He turned his back on Mr. Moore and walked down the hall.

Mr. Moore shrugged and returned to me. "See, I told you he wouldn't stay. He'll never change. He left A.M.A., and he'll leave again. Some of these guys just never appreciate what you do for them," he said and smiled sympathetically at me.

I realized suddenly that Mr. Moore, the guards, the rest of the staff, and all the patients I'd seen—everyone, that is, aside from Clint and me—were black. I started to wonder whether the hostility seeping around the edges of every encounter was abetted by something far deeper than Clint Wooder's fractiousness. Clint was white, and I was white, and those in charge were black. Could this be the anger of generations spilling over? I tasted—if only in a limited way—the powerlessness of the one excluded. I could feel the presence of unarticulated barriers, barriers I could never prove or even demonstrate, that would keep Clint from getting what I believed he needed. I would continue to do what I knew how to do, what usually worked in my middle-class, white world; but I realized then that there was nothing I could say or do that would change the outcome here. Things had already been decided.

The rest of the evening mirrored those first few minutes. I went down the empty hallway to the elevator, where Clint was smoking, to mollify him; and we turned back to the attendant. I asked to see the attending physician, who turned out to be an elderly white man standing just inside an open office door and trying unsuccessfully to interview a young black man sprawled in a chair, obviously spaced out on something. The physician hovered tentatively about the stuporous man, asking questions to which he received no answer, touching him timorously with his stethoscope now and then, maintaining physically what was an obvious emotional distance between his own world and the world of his patient. Receiving no answers, he left for his cubicle to write papers referring the young addict to the emergency room. I supposed—with not a little rancor—that the physician was retired, trying to earn a little extra by spending a few hours a week blessing with his title the process Clint and I had been experiencing. It was one more strike against the poor: With an occasional exception, only the least competent professionals stay in the front lines. Normally the work is left to those who long ago burned out.

I was allowed in to talk with the physician. "I'm Dr. Hedley," he said from behind his desk. He stood up and extended a thin hand. "Mr. Moore said you wanted to see me."

I introduced myself as a physician and mentioned my years of working with alcoholics and addicts. I told a bit about my personal connection with Clint, his six-month history of sobriety at Christ House, his relapse during the past two weeks, the frailty of his health in general, and his willingness to enter detox. "I've brought Mr. Wooder here for three days of detox; we'd be happy to take him back to Christ House after that."

Dr. Hedley smiled with strained politeness and studied the chart in front of him. "I see that Mr. Wooder left against medical advice the last time he was here. Mr. Moore informs me that there is a rule against admitting anyone who previously left A.M.A."

"The last time he was here was a year ago in January!" I said. "Are you saying that an alcoholic who once walks out of detox is forever banned from returning?"

Dr. Hedley looked down at the chart again. "Hmm, a year ago January . . . yes." He frowned. He paged idly through the chart, placed it carefully on the corner of his desk, lined up the corner of the chart precisely with the corner of the desk, and leaned back in his chair. "I'm sure you'd agree, Dr. Hilfiker, that it's very important to be firm with the addicted person. If one begins bending rules, one loses one's authority. I'm sure you know that from your experience. There are people in here who come in every weekend; I think they're probably after the meals. If one doesn't set limits, the system won't work. Don't you think so?" He smiled again and leaned forward in his chair.

"Dr. Hedley, Mr. Wooder hasn't been here in over twenty months; surely there's no rule against his admission."

He leaned back again and launched a long, rambling philosophical discourse about taxes and "firmness" and abuse of the system, but it was just smoke. The only public detoxification center in the city was refusing to accept an alcoholic relapsing after six months of sobriety, because he had walked away from the detox unit twenty months before.

When some months later I finally spoke to a physician in a position of authority within the Public Health Commissioner's office, he categorically denied that the city limited the availability of detox in any way. Detox was available to *anyone*, he assured me. I later confirmed this with the head of the alcohol and drug rehabilitation program. As often happens in the city—especially in regard to the poor, who have few advocates to fight for them—the *de facto* policy is considerably different from the *de jure* one.

Clint and I left a few minutes later. Clint was silent. I was the surprised and chastened one. I was running out of options that Clint knew he had run out of long ago. I drove Clint back to Christ House and—against all rules, rules I had long and loudly supported and strictly enforced, rules I had broken only for Scoop Miller—admitted him. To make matters worse, I knew Clint was returning to a staff divided in their feelings about him. Some of them, frightened by his sudden mood swings and the violence that had flared up several weeks earlier, would argue—as I had, other times, so vigorously—for strictness: "These are the rules; if you break them, you're out." Others, particularly the aides, had told me before almost bitterly that it was our rigidity that caused Clint's trouble in the first place. Admitting Clint would not be an easy solution.

I knew Clint would rebel. As he detoxed, he became more and more irritable, sullen, and uncooperative. I couldn't tell whether the staff's conflicting feelings showed, but I'm sure he sensed them, felt them as a kind of rejection. He kept asking me for higher doses of Librium, the tranquilizer I was using to detoxify him. I was again ambivalent. Aside from his irritability, he was showing few outward signs of withdrawal. I was already using more Librium than I had ever prescribed for anyone else, and I was afraid he was manipulating me into giving him drugs. Finally, I refused his requests point-blank. A few hours later he slammed out of the building, informing the nurses curtly that if we were not going to help him, he knew alcohol would quiet his nerves.

Though I despaired, I was frankly relieved that I didn't have to deal with Clint Wooder, at least for the moment. I was also angry at the hours of my personal time that Clint had sabotaged; angry at a private hospital refusing patients in need; angry at the city's alcohol treatment system and its staff full of people with chips on their shoulders; angry that there were—for the Clint Wooders of my world—no long-term treatment programs; angry even at the Christ House staff for wanting to enforce rules of which I had approved. It was as if Clint's agitation had rubbed off on me. I began feeling an almost global futility: Doesn't anyone get well? Am I just wasting my time? Clint was back on the street, and I was here. He would drink himself into the morgue, and I would go on to my next patient. What was the point?

But there were other feelings, too, ones I hardly recognized at the time. I was mourning the loss of a person I had come to treasure. I was experiencing, to some limited extent, Clint's helplessness, and it brought me a step closer to seeing the world from his point of view. I remembered my glib overconfidence several months earlier, when I had been sure Clint had made it after only a few months' sobriety. He hadn't accepted my reassurance. I recalled his respect for the abyss into which he'd now disappeared. And though I was afraid for him, I also felt a strange sense of privilege that Clint had shared part of his journey with me, that he had trusted me enough to show me his weakness as well as his strength.

Our relationship was not really a friendship based on reciprocity. Still, it was something meaningful forged in those small but crucial moments with another human being— moments of pain, weakness, failure, even heroism and success. Even as I mourned Clint, I knew he'd given me a gift. I felt more alive.

As a doctor I had little more to do with Clint, and I don't really know how the miracle occurred, only that it was a miracle. He survived his drunk and made it to the hospital once more. Eventually, he returned to the Samaritan Inn to begin again. Six months later I met him on the street. I felt that instant intimacy followed by hesitancy that one feels meeting an old high-school friend. He was still going to AA several times a day, and he still didn't know how long his sobriety would last, but he was finding new people in our community to support him in his life away from alcohol. Another day, I happened to talk with Clint's social worker at Samaritan Inn. The Angry had come back more than once, but Clint had weathered it. The next time I saw him, in front of Christ House, he told me about his new job as a part-time delivery person for a print shop downtown. A year later his employer—pleased with his work—hired him full-time. Clint moved into a small apartment of his own in the neighborhood, and he started returning to Christ House for our worship services.

It is Sunday morning, and Allen Goetcheus, pastor of the little congregation at Christ House, has chosen Clint to serve communion at our worship in the first-floor television room. As always, I am aware of the slightly acrid odor in the room, a thin film of cigarette tar covering the pale plaster walls. I take my place in the communion line, listening to the hymn in the background, vaguely noticing the scraping chairs as people stand and move. I try to reflect on the meaning of the Eucharist, but my attention focuses on Clint and the stone chalice in those dark, weathered hands. As I step toward him I look up, and he suddenly grins, a broad beaming smile, almost a laugh. Perhaps embarrassed, he catches himself and solemnly offers me the cup of communion, the laughter only in his eyes. "This is the blood of Jesus," he says, and I feel something crack within: All my awareness of the room and the other people and the hymn disappears. My vision blurs with tears, and I can feel my throat tightening. I give the chalice back and try to return his gaze, but I can't keep back the tears spilling down my cheeks.

The light covered by childhood abuse and drowned for so many years by alcohol has flickered and is now burning. I was Clint's companion on an important part of his journey, and I do not understand why he is even alive. How did he, who originally had no friends, no family, no work, nothing to look forward to even if he stayed sober, maintain a vision that sustained him through those dark days of recovery?

The years have passed. Clint Wooder has stayed sober. Every December he drops into our mailbox a Christmas card on which, in rough letters, he prints only his name; every spring, an Easter card. He lives in a basement apartment a few doors away, so we see each other on the street every month or two. We don't have much to say to one another, I suppose, but we usually stop and chat for a few minutes. Each of us seems to want to commemorate our experience together. Recently, Clint was laid off from the print shop, but he seems to be weathering this latest disappointment. Besides, his "mission work"—to talk to alcoholics on the street, help them get to detox, encourage them to enter treatment—is for him far more important. Clint remains for me a miracle, a reminder that there are events beyond our understanding, a sign of hope beyond despair.

Chapter 13

EPILOGUE

I have been here ten years now, between the worlds of the rich and the poor. And in truth, I'm not always sure what my presence has meant for these streets, for this community. My work puts me in daily contact with poor people, but the fog between us most often seems impenetrable. Friendship—as one might normally define it—has not been possible, and a real understanding of who my patients are has, I suspect, eluded me. Perhaps this is only my own personal weakness, the result of an inability to see empathically into a different culture . . . but I don't think so. I have come to believe that the worsening oppression of the poor and its consequent damage maintain this fog between us, fog so dense that we can, perhaps, never find our way through.

Suggs died recently of throat cancer. He had become my patient, and over the years in our many interactions I found him to be intelligent and knowledgeable, a man who read widely. Mathematically inclined, he supplemented his income doing taxes for others in the neighborhood. He took his antiseizure medicine regularly and periods of sobriety were fairly frequent. He still stopped in at the clinic twice a year for me to do a physical examination and fill out his GPA form, but I never felt I reached him in any meaningful way. As far as I know, he never dealt with his alcoholism;

251

in the last few years, he seemed somehow to have "burnt out." Even his death at D.C. General—the private hospital where his cancer was discovered refused him continuing care, and his referral to the public hospital was delayed over four months, by which time the cancer was beyond even palliative treatment—even his death testified to our abuse of the poor.

Delores Taylor and I have been in some limited sense reconciled since the day she came to the office for her disastrous GPA physical. I see her occasionally on the street and she greets me effusively as if I were an old and dear friend, but—though she still sometimes comes in to the office for prescription refills—she has never returned for another attempt at a physical examination. Another doctor—she isn't sure who or where—apparently convinced her to begin a new and much more effective regimen for her asthma, so her acute attacks are much less frequent.

David Lawson, remarkably, survives. His pancreatitis has subsided, so he no longer seems to have much abdominal pain. He stops by infrequently.

Many of the individuals I've written about here have disappeared from my life. I never saw Louise Flowers, Bernice Wardley, or Adelaid Beecher again. Margaret Mingo got tired of the trip across town, I suppose, and gradually stopped coming to the clinic, as did Marjawn Dixon. I've seen Scoop Miller just once in the last several years, when we met on the street. He looked fine and said he was working, but I have little idea how he really is, whether he stopped using, or where he may now be.

Many people have died. Jacinto Mendez was found dead on the street a block from Christ House. I was not surprised to hear that "One-Hand Joanne" had also died, without ever getting grafts for her skin ulcers. Apparently while in one of his depressions, Mr. Roberts committed suicide, and Mrs. Roberts died three years later in the hospital of a heart attack. Both were in their early forties.

The very poor have taken a particular battering in the last two decades. The undertow is powerful here in the inner city, overwhelming too many of those born into urban poverty, dragging away almost every chance for what the rest of us might call a "normal" life. A sober reading of our history does not leave much hope. There are more homeless and less housing. Children are born to damaged children. For every mother who courageously drags her children out of the despair, two, three, or four others are unable to escape their birth; anything that might make escape possible—adequate housing, basic education, jobs upon which one can support a family, accessible health care—is absent. By late 1992, I began to be unable to obtain needed referral care (specialists, testing, or hospitalization) for my patients even when I personally intervened. There is no breathing room left in the system; not even a middle-class advocate such as myself can get patients the care they need. society has given up, and no major figure of either political party as much as suggests plausible steps toward a possible restoration.

As I look around I find little to comfort me, even in the next generation. The children of the city are no longer simply the victims of violence and despair; they have also become the perpetrators. At Community of Hope, we have noticed that even our "own" children—those we have nurtured through summer youth programs and Sunday school—are selling drugs on the street corner, coming into the clinic with their beepers, dying in turf wars. Perhaps Shawn Baxter and Derwin Moseby are among them.

And then there is AIDS, only the most recent of the plagues to ravage the inner city. Despite our small size, over fifty Community of Hope patients are infected, among them Maggie Walker, the heroin addict who was so eager for help but for whom no program was available.

Yet in the midst of all this, despite the data that suggest its impossibility, I experience inexplicable hope. If I have learned anything, it is that many of the people with whom I work are heroes, people who struggle against all odds and survive; people who have been given less than nothing, yet find ways to give. An alcoholic of twenty years who has virtually nothing to return to suddenly stops using and becomes a force for health within the community. A homeless, single, unemployed mother with four children begins working as a receptionist in a social service agency and blossoms into a leader among other homeless mothers, providing hope, help, and inspiration. Women—many of them former alcoholics or drug addicts themselves—caring for the children of their cocaine-addicted daughters form a "grandmothers' group" to give one another emotional support and lobby (successfully) for changes in city regulations to allow them to receive the AFDC which would otherwise enable their daughters' drug use.

John Turnell has been sober over a year. When he last fell off the wagon, he'd been dry over fourteen months; his drunk lasted only a week. A disability determination through SSI finally came through, allowing him a monthly check for room and board. In 1993—as part of a new program for men who, though unlikely to be able to live independently anytime soon, were nevertheless maintaining sobriety—John, who was separated from his wife, moved into a third-floor guest room in Christ House to become a permanent member of the community. He is active in AA and has led others to sobriety. It is doubtful, I suppose, that he has seen his last drunk, but his periods of sobriety are getting longer, his drunks shorter. I think he will make it.

Although Kathy Bartlow has moved from Belmont Street and no longer comes to the clinic as a patient, she's visited several times. It's almost impossible to recognize her as the same woman to whom even the ambulance attendants refused care. She's been sober for several years, is back in touch with her children, and is working. I feel hopeful for her.

When I threw James Osborne out of Christ House because he couldn't stop drinking, he went back to the streets. Two years later he returned to Christ House with a large and ugly ulcer on his leg. But this time he was ready. He volunteered an interest in alcohol treatment and attended the twenty-eight-day program at Karrick Hall. I will not forget the Sunday he returned after his four weeks away. Allen Goetcheus asked him to read Scripture during the worship service at Christ House. Then, during communion, James sat deliberately on the far right end of the first row, where each person who took communion would have to pass. As each of us filed back to his seat, James reached and touched every one, hugging a few, shaking a hand or patting an elbow, welcoming us into fellowship with him, silently communicating how happy he was to be back. James, I think, will make it, too.

And I have moved on. First, in June 1990, Marja, the children, and I moved into a large, single-family dwelling we named Joseph's House; we invited eleven homeless men in the last stages of their struggles with AIDS to live out their days with us. Marja and I realized that we wanted to be closer to the people with whom we worked, that if we didn't move closer we might end up moving much farther away. To our surprise, our children were eager to make the change as well. Lois Wagner joined us as nurse, and a staff of about ten gradually came together, making possible round-the-clock care when necessary.

We lived as a community, sharing common space, eating together, gathering twice a week for meetings, and entering into the day-to-day routines of one another's lives. In those amazing, often chaotic three years, the coded locks came off the doors, the separate entrance disappeared, and we all lived in something more like the same place rather than simply in the same building. In those three years, an intimacy with those dying men became possible that, though still perhaps not a friendship as normally defined, was deeper than anything I'd ever experienced outside my family. The men who lived with me had to contend with my fears, limitations, and brokenness as much as, if not perhaps more than, I did with theirs.

Perhaps someday I will write a book about that, and about them. About Leroy—beaten as a child, sent to jail for murder in his early twenties, living for ten years in abandoned buildings as a "hopeless" alcoholic—who, though often cruel and sometimes devious, convinced me that the ability to experience joy and to trust can survive anything. About Clyde, an ex-burglar who lived for seventeen winters on the streets of Washington, who discovered through his incurable disease that the meaning of life lay in service to others. He dedicated his remaining years to giving his life away, volunteering at Mother Teresa's hospice for the destitute, where he accompanied homeless men dying of the same disease as his into their death, offering time and energy unstintingly to care for Joseph's House and its people. Or perhaps someone else will write that book. Or, as with almost everything else in the world of the poor, it may well be that those experiences will go unrecorded. Then no one will know of Walter's unremitting heroism in the face of his compulsive need for cocaine; of Manny's stubborn battle with his addiction, to the point that he incarcerated himself in the house for the last six months of his life to avoid temptation; of Tommy's unbearable hostility when he thought he'd been wronged and his profound humility when he realized his mistake. Whether or not their stories are publicly told, they have changed our lives forever.

In 1993, yet again demonstrating myself anything but a saint, I experienced my own version of burnout. Unlike John Turnell or Clint Wooder or Mrs. Mingo, however, I had a safety net—money, family, other work, a loving community to support me—and so I was able to retreat for a second year to Marja's home in Finland to recuperate. Where all this will lead me, I don't truly know; but never too far, I suspect, from the people of Belmont Street.

NOTES

1. It is true that over half of poor people in this country in 1989 were white, but *among* whites only 10 percent were poor, as opposed to 30.7 percent among blacks and 26.2 percent among Hispanics. See *Statistical Abstract of the United States 1989* (Washington, D.C.: U.S. Government Printing Office, 1989).
2. I have told this story in *Healing the Wounds: A Doctor Looks at His Work* (New York: Pantheon Books, 1985).
3. J. McAdam et al., "Tuberculosis in the SRO-Homeless Population," in *Health Care of Homeless People*, edited by P. Brickner et al. (New York: Springer Publishing, 1985), p. 170.
4. Michael Katz, *The Undeserving Poor* (New York: Pantheon Books, 1989), p. 187.
5. Fuller Torrey, Eve Barmann, and Sidney Wolfe, *Washington's Grate Society: Schizophrenia in the Shelters and on the Street* (Washington, D.C.: Public Citizen Health Research Group, 1985).
6. Ibid.
7. Ibid.
8. W. R. Breakey et al., "Health and Mental Problems of Homeless Men and Women in Baltimore," *Journal of the American Medical Association* 262 (1980): 1341–47.
9. Dorothy Wickenden, "Abandoned Americans," *New Republic*, March 18, 1985, pp. 19–25.
10. Katz, *Undeserving*, p. 189.
11. Center on Budget and Policy Priorities 1992 Report, as re-

.257

ported in *The Washington Post*, November 25, 1992, p. A8.
See also "Doubled-up Households in the District of Columbia," a report prepared by the Office of the Special Assistant
for Human Resource Development, Office of the Mayor
(1989).
12. Ibid.
13. The high-school-dropout rate in Washington, D.C., is not really known. In 1987 the "official" dropout rate (according to
the D.C. Public Schools Division of Quality Assurance) was
only 13.5 percent, but the method used to compute this figure
was blatantly deceptive. In 1984, 6,515 District of Columbia
students entered the tenth grade; three years later, only 3,715
had graduated, suggesting that approximately 2,800 dropped
out. This yields a dropout rate of 43 percent, the highest in
the nation. But—arguing that students who moved out of the
District shouldn't be counted as dropouts—city statisticians
subtracted from the 2,800 apparent dropouts the 1,916 students who (according to U.S. Census estimates) "might have
moved to another school district during this time." This left
only 884 dropouts. But having subtracted those who "might"
have moved away, those statisticians failed to add the approximately equal number of students who probably moved *into*
the District of Columbia in this period.
14. Katz, *Undeserving*.
15. See *No Room in the Marketplace: The Health Care of the
Poor*, Final Report of the Task Force on Health Care of
the Poor (St. Louis: Catholic Health Association, 1986).
16. Private health insurance has an administrative overhead of
about 14 percent, while Social Security and Medicaid (two
single-payer programs in the United States) average 3–4 percent. According to the General Accounting Office, a
Canadian-style single-payer system would save enough on
administrative overhead to cover all the uninsured and elimi-
nate all copayments and deductibles. From Steffie Wool-
handler, M.D., and David Himmelstein, M.D., "The Clinton
Plan: A Grim Fairytail," *Physicians for a National Health
Program Newsletter*, October 1993, pp. 3–10.
17. Ibid.